Archives of Animal Nutrition

Archiv für Tierernährung

VOLUME 37 · OCTOBER 1987 · NUMBER 10

AKADEMIE-VERLAG BERLIN

ISSN 0003-942X Arch. Anim. Nutr., Berlin 37 (1987) 10, 851–954

Archives of Animal Nutrition covers the following topics: Biochemical and physiological foundations of animal nutrition with emphasis laid on the following aspects: Protein metabolism, metabolism of non-protein-nitrogen compounds, energy transformation, mineral metabolism, vitamin metabolism, nutritional effects and performance criteria, furthermore: practical animal feeding, feedstuff theory, feedstuff preservation and feedstuff processing.

We accept for publication:

Original manuscript not yet published in other journals and not intended for publication in other journals in the same form. Their length should not exceed 12 printed pages.

Manuscripts are to be sent to Prof. HANS BERGNER, Wissenschaftsbereich Tierernährung der Sektion Tierproduktion und Veterinärmedizin, Humboldt-Universität zu Berlin, Invalidenstr. 42, DDR - 1040 Berlin. We request the authors to submit their manuscripts typed double-spaced and ready for print. The institution which the paper originates will be mentioned together with the author's name in the title of the paper.

The author is requested to discuss and summarize the results of his work at the end of the manuscript.

Author's names in the manuscript are to be underlined with a red wavy line. We request you to underline italics with a black or blue wavy line. Small print is to be indicated by a black or blue vertical line on the margin. Bibliographic data in the text are given with the name of the author and the year of publication, in case of several publications in one year, a, b, c etc. are added according to the sequence of the publications in the bibliography, e.g. MEYER (1985a). In the bibliography the papers are arranged alphabetically according to the name of the first author and quoted as follows: surname, first name, journal, volume, page and year.

Illustrations have to be restricted to the necessary minimum and to be enclosed separately. Indicative lines, letters etc. are to be entered in pencil. For photographes, a cover sheet should be used for this. The captions of the illustrations are to be listed on an extra sheet.

The authors receive 50 special prints of their contributions free of charge.

Terms of Subscription

Orders for the journal "Archives of Animal Nutrition" can be sent

- *in the GDR:* to the Postzeitungsvertrieb or to the Akademie-Verlag Berlin, Leipziger Str. 3–4, DDR - 1086 Berlin;
- *in the other socialist countries:* to a book-shop for foreign language literature or to the competent news-distributing agency;
- *in the FRG and Berlin (West):* to a book-shop or to the wholesale distribution agency Kunst und Wissen, Erich Bieber OHG, Wilhelmstr. 4–6, D - 7000 Stuttgart 1;
- *in the other Western European countries:* to Kunst und Wissen, Erich Bieber GmbH, General-Wille-Str. 4, Ch - 8002 Zürich;
- *in other countries:* to the international book- and journal-selling trade, to Buchexport, Volkseigener Außenhandelsbetrieb der DDR, Postfach 160, DDR - 7010 Leipzig, or to the Akademie-Verlag Berlin, Leipziger Str. 3–4, DDR - 1086 Berlin.

Zeitschrift „Archives of Animal Nutrition"

Herausgeber: Im Auftrag des Akademie-Verlages Berlin herausgegeben von Prof. Dr. Hans Bergner

Verlag: Akademie-Verlag Berlin, Leipziger Str. 3–4, DDR - 1086 Berlin.

Fernruf: 2 23 62 01 oder 2 23 62 29, Telex-Nr.: 11 44 20.

Bank: Staatsbank der DDR, Berlin Kto.-Nr.: 6836-36-20712.

Chefredakteur: Prof. Dr. sc. Hans Bergner.

Anschrift der Redaktion: Humboldt-Universität zu Berlin, Invalidenstr. 42, DDR - 1040 Berlin.

Veröffentlicht unter der Lizenznummer 1274 des Presseamtes beim Vorsitzenden
des Ministerrates der Deutschen Demokratischen Republik.

Gesamtherstellung: VEB Druckerei »Gottfried Wilhelm Leibniz«, DDR - 4450 Gräfenhainichen.

Erscheinungsweise: Archives of Animal Nutrition erscheint jährlich in einem Band mit zwölf Heften.

Bezugspreis je Band 360,– DM (zuzüglich Versandspesen); Preis je Heft 30,– DM.

Der gültige Jahresbezugspreis für die DDR ist der Postzeitungsliste zu entnehmen.

Bestellnummer dieses Heftes: 1010/37/10

AN (EDV) 39 532

02000

ARCHIVES OF ANIMAL NUTRITION
ARCHIV FÜR TIERERNÄHRUNG
VOLUME 37 · OCTOBER 1987 · NUMBER 10

Arch. Anim. Nutr., Berlin 37 (1987) 10, 851–859

Humboldt-University of Berlin, Department of Animal Nutrition (Head: Prof. Dr. sc. H. BERGNER)

O. SIMON, H. BERGNER and I. G. PARTRIDGE*

Estimation of the endogenous N proportions in ileal digesta and faeces in ^{15}N-labelled pigs

1. Introduction

Studies on protein digestion are complicated by the difficulty of distinguishing between undigested dietary N and endogenous N secreted into the digestive tract. Both of these components may be utilized by the bacteria in the large intestine to a greater or lesser degree. This problem has been studied in rats by labelling the dietary protein or the animal itself with ^{15}N (e.g. KRAWIELITZKI et al., 1977; BERGNER et al., 1978; SIMON et al., 1981; BERGNER & BERGNER, 1982; BERGNER et al., 1984; KÖHLER et al., 1984; PARTRIDGE et al., 1985). In the present trial an attempt was made to apply the technique of endogenous labelling with ^{15}N to the study protein digestion in pigs. At the same time the effects of increasing the dietary fibre content were studied by supplementation with treated straw meal. The effects of these treatments on the ileal and faecal digestibility of nutrients in the same study were presented by Partridge et al. (1986).

2. Methods

2.1. Animals

Four castrated male pigs were fitted with simple 'T' cannulas 30 cm cranial to the ileo-caecal junction under general anaesthetic. Their average weight during the experiment was approximately 40 kg.

* Animal and Grassland Research Institute, Shinfield, Reading, UK

2.2. ^{15}N labelling

After recovery from surgery the pigs were given ^{15}N-labelled ammonium salts orally for a period of 6 days. The compounds used were either $^{15}NH_4HCO_3$ (95 atom % excess, VEB Berlin Chemie, GDR) or a combination of this compound and $^{15}NH_4Cl$ (96 atom % excess, VEB Berlin Chemie, GDR) using equal proportions on an N basis. The amounts of ^{15}N given were based on metabolic body weight and were calculated to be 150 mg ^{15}N excess/$kg^{0.75}$/day.

The ^{15}N salts were added to a diet which consisted of wheat with mineral and vitamin supplements. This ensured a low dietary protein intake and therefore a high incorporation of non-specific N. The diet was restricted to 40 g/kg body weight per day, offered in two equal portions. The experimental levels of treated straw meal, as described below, were also introduced during the labelling period. Throughout the labelling period and the subsequent experimental period urine and faeces were collected daily in order to monitor ^{15}N excretion.

2.3. Experimental diets

During the trial itself the basal diet was composed of (g/kg): fish meal, 100; wheat, 880; mineral mixture, 10; vitamin mixture, 10. This was supplemented with varying levels of partially hydrolysed straw meal. Ground wheat straw was treated with HCl and steam, then neutralized with $Ca(OH)_2$, according to the method of BERGNER & BETZIN (1979). It was then dried and ground very finely.

The basal diet was given at a rate of 32 g/kg live weight/day in two equal portions. The experiment was divided into two periods of 5 days each during which the pigs received different supplements of straw meal. These supplements were such that the concentration of crude fibre in the diet ranged from 40 to 132 g/kg. Chromic oxide was added at a level of 5 g/kg of the complete diet. The chemical composition of the basal diet ingredients and straw meal have been given previously (PARTRIDGE *et al.*, 1986).

2.4. Digesta and faeces collection

During the last two days of each of the 5-day periods faeces were collected for 24 h, followed by 24 h digesta collections. Ileal digesta samples of ca. 700 g were obtained by fitting small polyethylene bags to the cannulas and collecting the contents each time the bags filled. The faeces and digesta samples were prepared for determination of chromic oxide and of the N and atom-% ^{15}N excess ($^{15}N'$) of TCA-soluble and TCA-precipitable fractions. Total N and $^{15}N'$ were determined by Kjeldahl digestion followed by steam distillation and titration of ammonia with HCl. The resulting samples were then dried and the atom-% $^{15}N'$ of the ammonium chloride was determined directly by emission spectrometry in an Isonitromat 5200 (VEB Statron, Fürstenwalde, GDR). Chromic oxide was assayed by the method of CHRISTIAN and COUP (1964).

At the end of the experiment, 14 days after the end of the labelling period, the pigs were slaughtered and various tissue samples were removed for $^{15}N'$ determinations, as described above.

3. Results and discussion

Fig. 1 shows the changes in atom-% ^{15}N excess in urine and faeces during the 6-day labelling period and throughout the experiment. After 1 or 2 days from the initiation of labelling, the ^{15}N abundance in urine reached a plateau. At the end of the labelling period there was a rapid decline in atom-% $^{15}N'$ until it reached a new plateau after

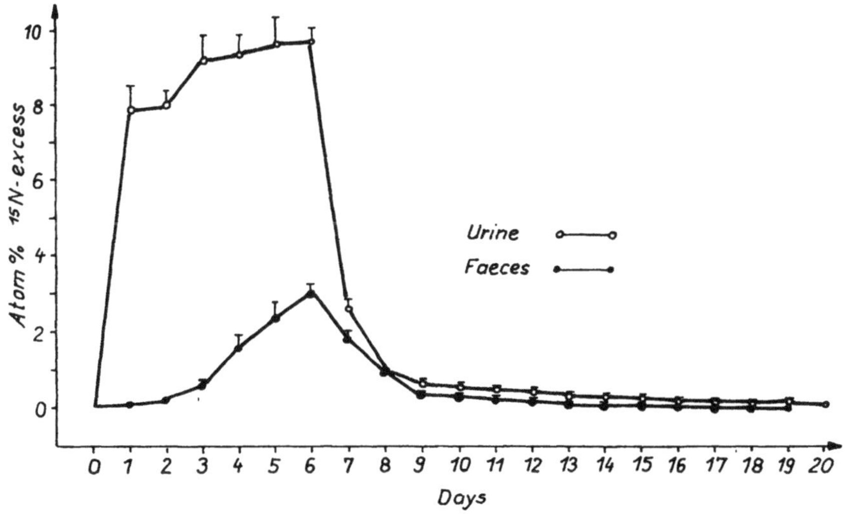

Fig. 1. Pattern of ^{15}N excretion in urine and faeces of pigs (Mean, SE of 3 animals) given ^{15}N ammonium salts. The label was given twice daily in the feed on days 1 to 6.

about 9 days from the start of the labelling period. Atom-% $^{15}N'$ in faeces followed a similar pattern but with a time lag of 1 to 2 days compared with urine, representing the intestinal transit of label secreted into the upper regions of the digestive tract. Four days after the oral doses of ^{15}N labelled compounds were withdrawn (10 days from the start) both urine and faeces ^{15}N abundance had reached a steady state and a constant ratio with each other. A very similar pattern of urine and faeces ^{15}N abundance was observed in rats given oral doses of ^{15}N labelled compounds by HERNÁNDEZ et al. (1981) and similar patterns of urine ^{15}N excretion in pigs were shown by BERGNER et al. (1984a).

The excretion of $^{15}N'$ in urine and faeces expressed as a proportion of the dose given during the 6-day labelling period is shown in Table 1. The values are given for only three animals because the fourth refused to consume the $^{15}NH_4Cl$ and therefore the time course of excretion and level of labelling were different. It is important to note that some individual pigs will not accept $^{15}NH_4Cl$ although all will readily consume $^{15}NH_4HCO_3$. The results presented in Table 1 show that 0.46 ± 0.058 of the dose was retained by the pigs. This shows the effectiveness of the labelling method which combined oral dosing with ^{15}N labelled salts and a low protein diet to ensure a high degree of incorporation of the label in body tissues. Similar conclusions were drawn in experiments with pigs by BERGNER et al. (1984a).

The atom-% ^{15}N excess in various body tissues following slaughter 14 days after the end of the labelling period are shown in Table 2, together with values for urine col-

Table 1

$^{15}N'$ excretion in pigs during a 6-day period in which they were given ^{15}N ammonium salts orally

Animal No.	$^{15}N'$ excretion as a proportion of intake		
	Urine	Faeces	Total
II	0.536	0.018	0.554
III	0.550	0.041	0.591
V	0.456	0.022	0.477

Animal No. VI was excluded from the table due to incomplete consumption of label

Table 2

Atom-% ^{15}N excess in various tissues and in urine two weeks after the end of oral labelling with ammonium salts (Mean ± SE from 4 pigs)

	Whole tissue homogenate	TCA-soluble fraction	TCA-precipitate fraction
Liver	0.31 ±0.021	0.24 ±0.017	0.32 ±0.022
Pancreas	0.28 ±0.015	0.31 ±0.019	0.29 ±0.011
Duodenum	0.22 ±0.014	0.22 ±0.014	0.21 ±0.008
Jejunum	0.19 ±0.013	0.21 ±0.019	0.20 ±0.003
Ileum	0.24 ±0.008	0.24 ±0.021	0.24 ±0.016
M. gastrocnemius	0.21 ±0.018	0.33 ±0.013	0.19 ±0.022
M. longissimus dorsi	0.19 ±0.030	0.33 ±0.047	0.19 ±0.026
Skin*	0.14 ±0.009	–	–
Urine**	0.22 ±0.011		

* Not homogenised

** Average for the last 3 days before slaughter

lected immediately before slaughter. There was good general agreement between the urine values and those for the TCA precipitable and TCA soluble fractions of tissue homogenates of the organs responsible for intestinal secretions. This indicates that it is valid to use the ^{15}N abundance in urine as an estimate of ^{15}N abundance in the endogenous secretions. Similar conclusions were drawn from comparisons of urine, blood and body tissue ^{15}N abundance in rats by SIMON et al. (1981). On this basis therefore, the endogenous components of ileal digesta and faeces were calculated according to the isotope dilution method proposed by KRAWIELITZKI & SMULIKOWSKA (1977):

$$\text{Endogenous N} = \frac{\text{atom-\% } ^{15}\text{N excess in total faeces or digesta}}{\text{atom-\% } ^{15}\text{N excess in endogenous N}}$$

using the urine atom-% ^{15}N excess as a measure of atom-% ^{15}N excess in endogenous N. In the case of faeces calculations a time lag of 24 h was allowed, to account for the transit of endogenous N compounds through the digestive tract.

As the ratio of ^{15}N excess in urine relative to faeces did not become stable until 6 days after the end of the labelling period (Fig. 1), it was not possible to calculate the endogenous N proportion in faeces until after this time. Hence the faeces data presented in Table 3 are for the second period of the trial only and are based on average

Table 3

Endogenous N as a proportion of total N in ileal digesta and faeces of pigs given various amounts of straw meal in the diet

Animal No.	Crude fibre content of diet (g/kg)	Endogenous proportion of N in Ileal digesta	Faeces[3]
II	40	0.491[1]	
VI	40	0.519[1]	
VI	40	0.435[2]	0.486
II	69	0.320[2]	0.439
V	83	0.361[1]	
V	100	0.300[2]	0.362
III	105	0.408[1]	
III	132	0.448[2]	0.382

[1] estimated on the fifth day after the end of the labelling period.
[2] estimated on the eleventh day after the end of the labelling period.
[3] average for the period from the sixth to the tenth day after the end of the labelling period.

values for urine and faeces during the period from the 6th to the 10th day after the end of the labelling period. Corresponding values are presented in Table 3 for digesta collected on days 5 and 11 after the end of the labelling period. Due to the relatively short transit time in the small intestine, the endogenous N component in digesta can be estimated rather sooner after the end of the labelling period than in faeces.

The endogenous N in ileal digesta ranged from 0.30 to 0.50 of total N and appeared to be independent of the level of crude fibre in the diet. In faeces the proportion of endogenous N was in the same range as that in ileal digesta, which suggests that both undigested dietary N and endogenous N reaching the large intestine are utilized by bacteria to a similar extent. In experiments with rats using the same method the endogenous proportion of N in faeces ranged from 0.50 to 0.60 (Hernández et al., 1981; Bergner et al., 1984b; Seidler et al., 1985). Using a different method, based on the comparative amino acid composition of digesta, diet and digestive secretions, Zebrowska et al. (1982) calculated that 0.50 to 0.60 of N passing through the terminal ileum of pigs was of endogenous origin. However, higher estimates of the endogenous proportion of N in faeces of rats have been reported (Bergner et al., 1978).

The total daily flow of N through the terminal ileum was calculated according to the chromic oxide ratio method. The average faecal N excretion was also determined for the 5 day balance period. Values for the endogenous proportions given in Table 3 were then applied, to calculate the absolute amounts of endogenous N and protein passing through the terminal ileum and excreted in faeces. These values, given in Table 4, showed no effect of the crude fibre content of the diet on endogenous N in ileal digesta. The average amount of endogenous protein passing through the terminal ileum was 21.4 g/day. This compares very well with the estimate of 21.9 g/day by Zebrowska et al. (1982) based on a completely different method (outlined earlier) in pigs of 33 kg given diets based on barley and soyabean meal.

Although the proportion of endogenous N in faeces was not affected by diet (Table 3) the total amount of N of endogenous origin excreted in faeces increased with in-

Table 4
Amounts of endogenous nitrogen and protein in ileal digesta and faeces of pigs given different amounts of straw meal in the diet

Animal No.	Crude Fibre content of diet (g/kg)	Endogenous nitrogen or protein (g) Ileal digesta N	Protein	Faeces N	Protein
II	40	3.90	24.4	–	–
VI	40	3.91	24.4	–	–
VI	40	2.96	18.5	1.35	8.44
II	69	3.22	20.1	1.36	8.50
V	83	2.75	17.2	–	–
V	100	3.24	20.2	2.11	13.2
III	105	2.90	18.1	–	–
III	132	4.56	28.5	1.92	11.97

creasing crude fibre intake (Table 4). The results in Table 4 also show clearly that about half of the endogenous protein which entered the large intestine was reabsorbed there.

Taking into account the estimated endogenous N content of ileal digesta a true ileal digestibility value of 0.83 ± 0.044 (s. d.) was calculated. This was 0.12 higher than the estimated apparent digestibility. Similarly, the overall apparent and true digestibilities were calculated, on the basis of faecal measurements. These decreased from 0.91 and 0.96 respectively for the basal diet to 0.83 and 0.89 respectively for the highest dietary crude fibre level.

It was calculated that in ileal digesta 0.55 ± 0.113 of the total N was in the TCA precipitable fraction, compared with 0.43 ± 0.114 of the endogenous N. These compare favourably with values of 0.56 and 0.37 respectively for the TCA precipitable fractions of total and endogenous N in the distal small intestine in rats (PARTRIDGE et al., 1985). This seems to suggest that residual dietary protein in the lower small intestine is of low digestibility, probably due to its association with the fibre fractions of the diet ingredients. In faeces 0.89 ± 0.035 of total N was in the TCA precipitable fraction compared with 0.87 ± 0.058 of the N of endogenous origin.

4. Conclusions

By feeding a low protein diet it was possible to achieve a retention of ^{15}N labelled non-specific N which approached half of the dose given as ammonium salts. A good agreement between the ^{15}N abundance in urine and secretory organs demonstrated the validity of using urine values as a measure of ^{15}N abundance in endogenous N. The average amount of endogenous N passing the terminal ileum was 3.4 g/day and was not affected by dietary fibre level. This represented 0.30 to 0.50 of total ileal N flow. The proportion of faecal N which was of endogenous origin was similar to that in ileal digesta, suggesting similar utilization of endogenous and undigested dietary N by large intestine bacteria. Half of the endogenous N entering the large intestine was reabsorbed there. Increasing the crude fibre content of the diet from 40 to 132 g/kg increased the quantity of endogenous N in the faeces from about 1.3 to 2.0 g/day.

Summary

Four 40 kg castrated male pigs fitted with simple 'T' cannulas in the terminal ileum were given ^{15}N-labelled ammonium salts, added to a low protein diet, for 6 days. Excretion of ^{15}N in urine and faeces was monitored daily throughout the labelling and subsequent experimental periods. During the experimental period the pigs were given a diet based on wheat and fish meal, supplemented with varying levels of partially hydrolysed straw meal to give crude fibre contents ranging from 40 to 132 g/kg. After adaptation to the particular levels of straw meal, faeces and ileal digesta were collected during successive 24 h periods. N digestibility values were determined by the chromic oxide ratio method. The retention of ^{15}N labelled non-specific N was 0.46 of the dose given. The validity of using urine values as a measure of ^{15}N abundance in endogenous N was demonstrated by the similarity of ^{15}N abundance in urine immediately before slaughter at the end of the experiment and in the digestive secretory organs thereafter. The average amount of endogenous N passing the terminal ileum was 3.4 g/day or 0.30–0.50 of total ileal N flow. This was not affected by dietary fibre level. The proportion of faecal N which was of endogenous origin was similar to that in ileal digesta, suggesting similar utilization of endogenous and residual dietary N by hindgut bacteria. Half the endogenous N entering the large intestine was reabsorbed there. Increasing dietary crude fibre from 40 to 132 g/kg increased faecal endogenous N excretion from 1.3 to 2.0 g/animal and day.

Zusammenfassung

O. Simon, H. Bergner und I. G. Partridge

Ermittlung des endogenen N-Anteils in der ilealen Digesta und im Kot von ^{15}N-markierten Schweinen

Vier Börge (LM 40 kg), die mit einfachen „T"-Fisteln im terminalen Ileum versehen waren, erhielten 6 Tage lang ^{15}N-Ammoniumsalze, die einer Diät mit niedrigem Proteingehalt zugesetzt wurden. Während der Markierungsperiode und den darauffolgenden Versuchsperioden wurde die ^{15}N-Ausscheidung mit Harn und Kot täglich ermittelt. Während der Versuchsperiode erhielten die Schweine eine Diät, die auf Weizen und Fischmehl basierte und die mit verschiedenen Mengen teilhydrolysiertem Strohmehl supplementiert war, so daß sich Rohfasergehalte von 40 bis 132 g/kg ergaben. Nach Adaption an die entsprechende Strohmehlgabe wurden Kot und Ileumdigesta aufeinanderfolgend je 24 Std. gesammelt. Die N-Verdaulichkeitswerte wurden mit der Cr_2O_3-Methode ermittelt.

Die Retention von ^{15}N-markiertem unspezifischem N betrug 46 % der verabreichten Dosis. Die Möglichkeit, Harn-N-Werte als Maß für die ^{15}N-Häufigkeit des endogenen N zu verwenden, wurde anhand der ähnlichen ^{15}N-Häufigkeit im Harn unmittelbar vor der Schlachtung und den sekretorischen Verdauungsorganen, nachgewiesen. Im Durchschnitt passierten 3,4 g endogener N/Tag das terminale Ileum, was 30–50 % des gesamten ilealen N-Flusses ausmachte. Diese Werte wurden nicht durch den Rohfasergehalt der Ration beeinflußt. Der N-Anteil endogenen Ursprungs im Kot war ebenso groß wie in der Ileumdigesta, was auf eine gleiche Verwertung von endogenem und von restlichem Diät-N durch Dickdarmbakterien hinweist. Die Hälfte des in den Dickdarm gelangenden endogenen N wurde dort rückresorbiert. Die Erhöhung des Rohfaseranteils in der Diät von 40 auf 132 g/kg führte zu einer Erhöhung der fäkalen Exkretion an endogenem N von 1,3 auf 2,0 g/Tier · d.

Резюме

О. Симон, Х. Бергнер и И. Г. Партридж

Определение эндогенной доли азота в содержимом илеума и в кале у меченых ^{15}N свиней

4 борова (40 кг ЖМ), имеющих простые анастомозы вида «Т» у терминального илеума, получили в течение 6 дней соли ^{15}N-аммония, которые добавились к диете с низким содержанием протеина. Во время периода мечения и последовательских опытных периодов определилось суточное выделение ^{15}N с мочой и калом. Во время опытного периода свиньи получили диету, которая базировалась на пшенице и рыбной муке. К этой диете добавились различные количества частично гидролизированной соломенной муки, таким образом получились содержания клетчатки от 40 до 132 г/кг. После адаптации к соответствующей даче соломенной муки собрались друг за другом кал и содержимое илеума, каждый за 24 часа. Переваримость азота определилась с помощью индикатора Cr_2O_3.

Ретенция неспецифического и меченого ^{15}N азота составила 46 % от введенной дозы. Данные содержания N в качестве для частоты ^{15}N эндогенного азота можно пользоваться, что показало определение подобной частоты ^{15}N в моче непосредственно до убоя и в секреторных пищеварительных органах.

В среднем определились в сутки 3,4 г эндогенного азота как пассаж через терминальный илеум, что было 30–50 % общего илеального пассажа N. Эти данные не зависили от содержания клетчатки рациона. Доля эндогенного N в кале была равной доли эндогенной N содержимого илеума, что ссылает на равное использование эндогенного и остаточного из диеты N бактериями толстой кишки. Половина эндогенного N, вводившегося в толстую кишку, здесь обратно всасывалась. Повышение содержания клетчатки в диете от 40 до 132 г/кг вело к повышению выделения эндогенного N с калом от 1,3 до 2,0 г на голову в сутки.

References

[1] BERGNER, U., K. ADAM and H. BERGNER: Arch. Tierernähr. **28**, 585 (1978)
[2] BERGNER, U. and H. BERGNER: Arch. Tierernähr. **32**, 841 (1982)
[3] BERGNER, H., U. BERGNER and K. ADAM: Arch. Tierernähr. **34**, 441 (1984a)
[4] BERGNER, H. and B. BETZIN: Arch. Tierernähr. **29**, 119 (1979)
[5] BERGNER, H., W. SEIDLER, O. SIMON and H. SCHMANDKE: Ann. of Nutr. and Metabol. **28**, 156 (1984b)
[6] CHRISTIAN, K. R. and M. R. COUP: New Zealand J. of Sci. and Technol. A, **36**, 328 (1964)
[7] HERNÁNDEZ, M., O. SIMON and H. BERGNER: Arch. Tierernähr. **31**, 651 (1981)
[8] KÖHLER, R., T. PAHLE and G. GEBHARDT: Arch. Tierernähr. **34**, 111 (1984)
[9] KRAWIELITZKI, K. and S. SMULIKOWSKA: Arch. Tierernähr. **27**, 39 (1977)
[10] KRAWIELITZKI, K., T. VÖLKER, S. SMULIKOWSKA, H.-D. BOCK and J. WÜNSCHE: Arch. Tierernähr. **27**, 609 (1977)

[11] PARTRIDGE, I. G., O. SIMON and H. BERGNER: Arch. Tierernähr. **35**, 163 (1985)
[12] PARTRIDGE, I. G., O. SIMON and H. BERGNER: Arch. Tierernähr. **36**, 353 (1986)
[13] SEIDLER, W., H. BERGNER, O. SIMON and H. SCHMANDKE: Ann. of Nutrit. and Metabol. **29**, 184 (1985)
[14] SIMON, O., M. HERNÁNDEZ and H. BERGNER: Arch. Tierernähr. **31**, 739 (1981)
[15] ZEBROWSKA, T., O. SIMON, R. MÜNCHMEYER, E. WOLF, H. BERGNER and H. ZEBROWSKA: Arch. Tierernähr. **32**, 431 (1982)

The authors thank Dr. H. ROHRMANN for assistance with the surgery, Mrs. B. BETZIN for preparation of the straw meal, Mrs. I. BECKER, Mrs. I. DRESSEL, Mr. K.-P. GÖTZ, Mrs. U. KITTLER and Mrs. S. KIEWEL for technical assistance.

Received 17 April 1986

Address of authors:

Prof. Dr. sc. H. BERGNER and Dr. sc. O. SIMON
Humboldt-University of Berlin
Department of Animal Nutrition
Invalidenstr. 42
Berlin
DDR - 1040

Dr. I. G. PARTRIDGE
Heritage Gate. Friary Street
Derby DE 1 1QR
UK

Arch. Anim. Nutr., Berlin 37 (1987) 10, 860

Buchbesprechung

Rindfleischproduktion (Production de Viande Bovine), Herausgeber: D. Micol

Erschienen im Institut National de la Recherche Agronomique, Paris, 1986, 504 Seiten, 186 Tab., 126 Abb., Format 15×24, kartoniert, Preis 185,– FF.

Seit mehr als 15 Jahren organisiert das Forschungszentrum für Zootechnik und Veterinärwesen des französischen Nationalinstitutes für Landwirtschaftsforschung (INRA) in Theix Jahrestagungen zu ausgewählten Problemen der Tierproduktionsforschung. Die XV. Tagung, die in der Zeit vom 5.–7. Juni 1984 stattfand, befaßte sich mit dem Themenkomplex Rindfleischproduktion und führte Wissenschaftler aus den verschiedensten einschlägigen Forschungseinrichtungen Frankreichs und Spezialisten der Produktion, der Verarbeitungsindustrie und des Vermarktungssektors zusammen. Im vorliegenden Buch hat der Herausgeber Didier Micol, wissenschaftlicher Mitarbeiter am Laboratorium für Fleischproduktion des INRA in Theix, die im Verlauf der Veranstaltung gehaltenen Referate sowie die Hauptinhalte der Rundtischgespräche zusammengestellt. In vier Schwerpunkten gegliedert, wird dem Leser ein umfassender Überblick über den gegenwärtigen Stand der Forschungen auf dem Gebiet der Rindfleischproduktion in Frankreich und damit gleichzeitig ein Zeugnis der zielstrebigen komplexen Bearbeitung dieser Thematik, insbesondere durch Wissenschaftler des INRA, gegeben. In zwölf Vorträgen werden sowohl physiologische, genetische, nährstoffökonomische, technologische und finanzielle Aspekte der Produktion von Rindfleisch beleuchtet. So setzen sich die Autoren mit Problemen der Schlachtkörperzusammensetzung und der Qualität des Rindfleisches auseinander, stellen Ergebnisse der genetischen Verbesserung des Tiermaterials vor, vergleichen unterschiedliche Richtungen und Verfahren der Rindfleischproduktion, behandeln die damit im Zusammenhang stehenden ökonomischen Probleme und geben letztlich einen Ausblick auf Entwicklungstendenzen der Konsumtion und Vermarktung.

Aus der Sicht der Tierernährung bzw. Tierfütterung sind die Ausführungen zu unterschiedlichen Fütterungsregimen und Rationstypen unter weitestgehender Nutzung von Grobfutterstoffen (Gras und Grünmais bzw. deren Silagen) von besonderem Wert.

Umfangreiches Zahlenmaterial, verständlich gestaltete Tabellen und Abbildungen untermauern die getroffenen Aussagen. Jedem Vortrag sind in unterschiedlichem Umfang Literaturangaben zugeordnet.

Als nützlich und informativ werden auch die im letzten Kapitel des Buches resumeartig dargelegten Hauptgedanken der fünf Rundtischgespräche angesehen. Zwei dieser Gesprächsrunden waren Problemen der Tierernährung im Zusammenhang mit der Rindfleischproduktion gewidmet. Von Interesse sind neben den Angaben zur Energie-, Nährstoff- und Mineralstoffversorgung die neuen Ergebnisse zum Einsatz von Futterzusatzstoffen, insbesondere von Anabolika.

Auf Grund seiner Komplexität spricht das Buch einen breiten Interessentenkreis an, der nicht nur Wissenschaftler und Spezialisten der Tierproduktion umfaßt. Wertvolles Gedankengut ist dem Buch auch vom Fachmann der Lebensmittelindustrie, insbesondere der Fleischverarbeitung und -vermarktung, zu entnehmen.

W.-B. Souffrant

Arch. Anim. Nutr., Berlin 37 (1987) 10, 861–867

Institute of Animal Physiology and Nutrition
Polish Academy of Sciences, Jablonna near Warsaw, Poland
(Director Prof. Dr. S. BURACZEWSKI)[1]
Institute of Animal Nutrition, FAL
Bundesallee 50, D - 3300 Braunschweig, F.R. Germany
(Director Prof. Dr. H. J. OSLAGE)[2]

LUCYNA BURACZEWSKA[1], E. SCHULZ[2] and HARRIET SCHRÖDER[2]

Ileal digestibility of amino acids in pigs fed barleys differing in protein content

1. Introduction

Barley provides a large proportion of dietary protein for pigs in many countries. Its proteins are deficient in some amino acids therefore an accurate knowledge of amino acid digestibility is of practical importance for correct supplementation of cereal–based diets with amino acids of synthetic or protein origin. Barley varies widely in total protein content and its digestibility. SCHULZ and OSLAGE (1969) in their investigations on nutritive value of different home-grown and foreign barleys found a positive correlation between the crude protein content and its digestibility in pigs. EGGUM (1973) reviewed many studies and found that the variation in protein and amino acid digestibility of barley was related both to protein and to its tannin content. Since many years it has been generally recognized as important to estimate ileal rather than faecal digestibility of amino acids in feedstuffs as a measure of their availability to pigs. Faecal analysis method has been often criticized because of possible microbial alterations of undigested and unabsorbed nitrogenous residues in the large intestine (CHO et al., 1971; ŻEBROWSKA, 1973; ŻEBROWSKA et al., 1978; JUST et al., 1981). The results published up to now show large differences concerning ileal digestibility of nutritionally important amino acids of barley. For example the values given for lysine apparent digestibility at the ileal level range from 65 (SAUER et al., 1981) to 79 per cent (JUST et al., 1981). The question arises whether and to what extent the ileal digestibility values are influenced by crude protein and fibre content of the grain. Since experiments to obtain digestibility values are costly and require much time and effort the further research goals should be to predict amino acid digestibility from nitrogen digestibility or other indices.

The aim of this study was to determine the apparent digestibility of protein and amino acids at the terminal ileum and over the entire digestive tract of growing pigs fed barley differing in nitrogen content.

2. Materials and methods

Male pigs in the range of live weight from 28 to 76 kg with simple cannula in the terminal ileum were fed with diets of nine different barleys (Table 1) as the only feed. The diets were supplemented with vitamins and minerals and chromium oxide was added

Table 1

Dry matter (DM) content and chemical characteristics of barleys (amino acids in g/16 g N; other substances in per cent of DM)

No*	1	2	3	4	5	6	7	8	9
Variety	Grit	Aramir	Gunhild** Georgie	Diva	Aramir	Ingri** Tapir Sonia	Aramir	Diva	Ingri** Tapir
DM	88.9	89.0	89.7	87.6	89.4	89.0	88.3	87.5	89.3
N	1.73	1.80	1.88	1.98	2.00	2.01	2.05	2.10	2.16
NDF	13.82	13.93	16.61	13.45	14.06	13.89	15.57	14.85	15.52
ADF	5.87	5.32	6.06	5.32	5.00	5.29	6.45	5.53	5.41
Hemicel-lulose	7.95	8.61	10.55	8.13	9.06	8.60	9.12	9.32	10.11
Crude fibre	4.85	4.74	5.19	4.36	4.79	4.59	5.20	5.24	4.91
Lys	3.82	3.79	3.66	3.63	3.67	3.47	3.50	3.53	3.26
Cys	2.29	2.11	2.09	2.12	2.23	2.10	2.13	2.08	2.15
Met	1.93	1.93	1.78	1.74	1.81	1.74	1.80	1.81	1.86
Trp	1.27	1.15	1.17	1.18	1.21	1.22	1.20	1.22	1.27
Thr	3.51	3.58	3.46	3.43	3.50	3.37	3.45	3.47	3.38
Ile	3.60	3.54	3.68	3.47	3.58	3.48	3.50	3.55	3.51
Val	5.12	5.02	5.21	4.85	4.98	4.82	5.00	4.69	4.86
Leu	6.61	6.86	7.06	6.44	6.60	6.44	6.54	6.52	6.84
His	2.22	2.19	2.20	2.15	2.16	2.14	2.21	2.13	2.09
Phe	4.94	5.09	5.18	4.92	5.09	5.26	5.05	5.11	5.41
Arg	5.30	5.26	5.27	4.87	4.98	4.67	4.95	4.83	4.73

* Nos 1, 2, 3, 4, 5, 7 and 8 were summer barleys and no 6 and 9 winter barleys
** Mixture of two or three varieties

They were fed according to body weight (with age, from 4.3 to 3.8 per cent b. w.) for 12 days, each to 4, 5 or 6 pigs. The diets were offered in the wet form in two meals given every 12 h.

After 6 days of preliminary period, faeces were collected for 72 h from the seventh to the ninth day and digesta for three 12 h periods from the tenth to the twelfth day by using plastic tube. Faeces and digesta were freeze-dried and pooled samples were prepared for total collection period of digesta (36 h) from each pig on dry matter basis.

Chromium content was determined by a method based on that described by PETRY and RAPP (1970/71). Fibre fractions NDF and ADF were analyzed according to Fibertec System M using the method developed by VAN SOEST ("Tecator", Application note). Samples for NDF determination were incubated with amylase after detergent treatment to remove the rest of starch from the crucible remaining. Amino acids were analysed with Beckman analyzer.

3. Results and discussion

The contents of nitrogen, amino acids and fibre fractions in different barleys are presented in Table 1. Within the barleys the amount of lysine decreased from 3.82 to 3.26 g/16 g N as the N content increased from 1.73 to 2.16 per cent/DM. Acid- and neutral-detergent fibre appeared not to be closely related indicating a variable content (from 8.0 to 10.6 %) of hemicellulose, calculated by difference between the NDF and ADF values. This fact is in agreement with observations made by TAVERNER and FARRELL (1981 b) on wheats. However, the authors found a negative correlation between nitrogen content of barley and its hemicellulose content. In contrast the nitrogen content of wheat was positively correlated with all fibre fractions.

Fig. 1 shows the results of apparent ileal digestibility of crude protein related to nitrogen content of eight barleys (excluding No. 9). The regression coefficient of the linear regression equation ($r = 0.87$) was positive and statistically significant. This is

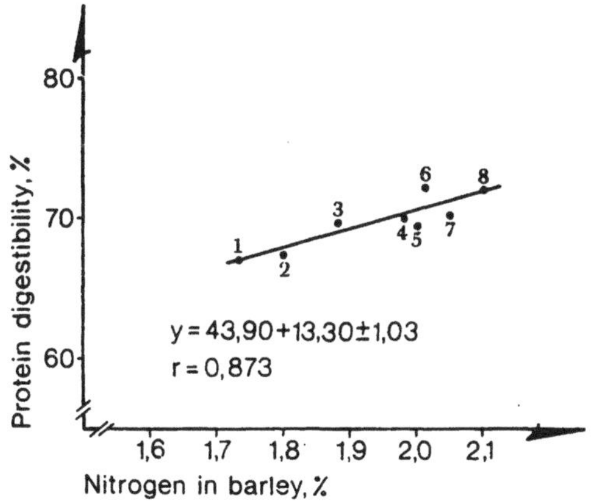

Fig. 1. Relationship between app. ileal digestibility of protein and nitrogen level in eight barleys (nos 1–8)

in agreement with SCHULZ and OSLAGE (1969) and EGGUM (1973) who reported a positive relationship between the digestibility and the content of protein in barley. Generally, the higher the protein content in the grain the higher the apparent amino acid digestibility measured at the ileum. However, in our case the digestibilities for barley no 4 were somewhat higher than that of nos 5 and 7, and that of no 6 higher than that of nos 7 and 8, what was probably due to comparatively lower NDF content in barleys nos 4 and 6. There are many evidences that cell wall carbohydrates may be a factor affecting protein digestibility and amino acid availability of a diet (FERNANDEZ and JØRGENSEN, 1986).

Another possible reason for the observed differences between the barleys could be due to differences in the relative and absolute proportions of each of the four major protein fractions of barley (albumin, globulin, glutelin and prolamin) which differ in amino acid composition and are dependent on the variety and environmental conditions under which these are grown (SODEK and WILSON, 1971; ABROL et al., 1971). Since a substancial proportion of albumin and globulin protein in grains is contained in aleurone cells, which in barley has a multicellular cell layer (POSTEL, 1957), it can perhaps influence digestibility as these cells are not efficiently broken down because of their thick cellulosic cell wall (SAUNDERS et al., 1969). These observations are in agreement with BACH-KNUDSEN et al. (1982) finding that the high lysine barley var. M-1508 contained in endosperm more β-glucans and hemicellulose than the normal mother var. Bomi. It was assumed that this was a reason of the lower values for the protein digestibility and digestible energy of endosperm from M-1508 compared to the values for Bomi.

The average values for ileal and faecal apparent digestibilities are presented in Fig. 2. The graph shows that for nitrogen as well as for most of the amino acids the faecal values were greater than the ileal ones. In the case of nitrogen the average faecal value exceeded in about 10 digestibility units what is in the range (from 8 to 15) observed by

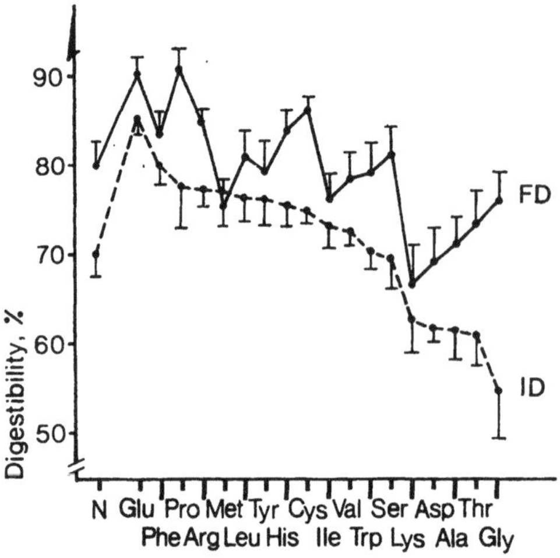

Fig. 2. App. ileal (ID) and faecal (FD) digestibility of amino acids in pigs fed eight barleys (average values with standard deviation)

other authors (SAUER et al., 1977, 1981; TAVERNER and FARRELL, 1981 a; ŻEBROWSKA et al., 1984; JUST et al., 1981; POPPE et al., 1983). Among the dispensible amino acids, glycine, proline and serine disappeared to the largest extent in the large intestine. What the nutritionally more important amino acids is concerned, for cystine, valine, histidine, tryptophan and threonine faecal analysis originates overestimation ranging from 6 to 12 units and less for other amino acids. For methionine the faecal as compared to ileal digestibility value indicates even a net increase which is consistent with the results reported by many authors (CHO and BAYLEY, 1972; JUST et al., 1980; TAVERNER and FARRELL, 1981 d; ŻEBROWSKA et al., 1984) and not only for grains but also for other feedstuffs. The differences of individual amino acids in the large intestine is thought to be primarily due to bacterial fermentation and synthesis in this part of the digestive tract. As the bacterial processes depend on the availability of nitrogen and energy, the differences between faecal and ileal values were somewhat smaller for the higher digestible barleys which contained more than 2 per cent N and less than 12 per cent NDF.

When comparison was made between the ileal amino acid and nitrogen digestibilities, which can be predicted from the equation given in Fig. 1, the value for tryptophan was similar to that of nitrogen, for lysine and threonine being 7–8 digestibility units lower, for isoleucine and valine 2–3 units higher, for cystine, histidine, leucine and methionine 5–6 units higher and in the case of phenylalanine even up to 10 digestibility higher than the value for nitrogen. As it is shown of the indispensable amino acids in barley, the recoveries of lysine and threonine, the most limiting amino acids in barley protein, were approximately equal in being the lowest at the end of the ileum what is consistent with findings for five different cultivars by SAUER et al. (1977, 1981) and with those given for one barley by TAVERNER et al. (1981). In later work on nutritive value of barley for pigs (TAVERNER et al., 1982) the authors suggest that for practical purposes the digestible lysine content of barley can be calculated using an average value for lysine digestibility of 77 per cent. This is much higher than our value (av. 70 %) or those found by SAUER et al., 1981 (av. 70 %) and by POPPE et al., 1983 (69 %).

JUST et al. (1983) studied possibilities for prediction of the feed value of four variety of barley on the basis of easy measurable properties such as density, kernel weight and chemical components. Statistical analysis of the values showed only small correlations and poor possibility for the prediction unless a large number of variables are included in the prediction equation. However, the content of digestible crude protein and digestible lysine as well as of the protein deposition was significantly improved by extra nitrogen fertilization of spring barley and wheat.

Summary

The apparent digestibility of nitrogen and amino acids was measured by the ileal and faecal methods in pigs fed nine barleys differing in nitrogen content (from 1.73 to 2.16 per cent/DM). A positive ($r = 0.87$) and significant relationship was found between the apparent nitrogen digestibility at the end of the ileum and the crude protein content of barley. Generally, the higher the protein of the grain, the higher the ileal digestibilities of the amino acids. For most amino acids the faecal values were greater than the ileal ones. This being specially so for threonine, tryptophan, histidine and cystine belonging to the nutritionally important amino acid group. When the relationship between the amino acid and nitrogen digestibilities at the level of ileum is considered, the values were found to be similar to that of nitrogen in the case of tryptophan, higher for isoleucine, valine (both 2–3 units), cystine, histidine, leucine, methionine (all 5–6 units) and phenylalanine (10 units) and lower only for lysine and threonine (7–8 dig. units).

Zusammenfassung

LUCYNA BURACZEWSKA, E. SCHULZ und HARRIET SCHRÖDER

Ileale Verdaulichkeit von Aminosäuren bei Schweinen nach Verfütterung von Gersten unterschiedlichen Proteingehaltes

Es wurde die scheinbare Verdaulichkeit von Stickstoff und Aminosäuren bei Schweinen am Illeumende und im Kot nach Verfütterung von neun Gersten mit unterschiedlichen Stickstoffgehalten bestimmt (von 1,73 bis 2,16 % N i. TS). Zwischen der scheinbaren Stickstoffverdaulichkeit am Ende des Illeums und dem Rohproteingehalt der Gerste bestand eine signifikante, positive Beziehung ($r = 0{,}87$). Allgemein stieg die ileale Verdaulichkeit der Aminosäuren mit zunehmendem Proteingehalt des Getreides an. Für die meisten Aminosäuren konnten höhere fäkale als ileale Werte gefunden werden. Dies traf für die essentiellen Aminosäuren Threonin, Tryptophan, Histidin und Zystin zu. Ein Vergleich der Verdaulichkeitswerte zwischen Aminosäuren und Stickstoff am terminalen Ileum ergab übereinstimmende Werte für Tryptophan, höhere für Isoleuzin, Valin (jeweils 2–3 Einheiten), Zystin, Histidin, Leuzin, Methionin (alle 5–6 Einheiten) und Phenylalanin (10 Einheiten) und niedrigere Werte nur für Lysin und Threonin (7–8 Einheiten).

Резюме

Люцина Бурачевска, Е. Шульц и Харриет Шрёдер

Переваримость аминокислот определяемая в конце бедренной кишки у свиней кормленных ячменем с разным содержанием протеина

Видимая переваримость азота и аминокислот определяли в конце бедренной кишки и в кале свиней кормленных девяти сортами ячменя с разным содержанием азота (от 1,73 до 2,16 % сухого вещества). Установили положительную ($r = 0,87$) и достоверную взаимосвязь между кажущуюся переваримостью азота в конце бедренной кишки и содержанием сырого протеина в ячмене. В общем чем больше протеина в зерне, тем выше коэффициенты переваримости аминокислот. Для большинства аминокислот коэффициенты определенные в бедренной кишке нисшие чем измеренные в кале. Это относится особенно к треонину, триптофану, гистидину и цистину принадлеждящих к группе аминокислот важных для питания животных. Если рассматривать взаимосвязь между переваримостью аминокислот и азота на уровне бедренной кишки величины найдены для триптофана были подобные как для азота, высшие для изолейцина, валина (обеих на 2–3 единицы коэффициентов переваримости), цистина, гистидина, лейцина (всех на 5–6 единиц) и фенилаланина (10 единиц), и нисшие только для лизина и треонина (7–8 единиц).

References

[1] Abrol, Y. P., D. C. Uprety, U. P. Ahiya and M. S. Naik: Aust. J. Agric. Res. **22**, 195 (1971)
[2] Bach-Knudsen, K. E., J. Wolstrup and B. O. Eggum: J. Anim. Physiol. a. Anim. Nutr. **48**, 276 (1982)
[3] Cho, C. Y. and H. S. Bayley: Can. J. Physiol. Pharmac. **50**, 513 (1972)
[4] Cho, C. Y., F. D. Horney and H. S. Bayley: Fed. Proc. **30**, 235 (1971)
[5] Eggum, B. O.: A study of certain factors influencing protein utilisation in rats and pigs Rolighedsveg 26, 1958-København V. (1973)
[6] Fernandez, J. A. and H. Jørgensen: Liv. Prod. Sci. **15**, 53 (1986)
[7] Just, A., H. Jørgensen and J. A. Fernandez: Br. J. Nutr. **46**, 209 (1981)
[8] Just, A., H. Jørgensen, J. A. Fernandez and H. M. Jepsen: Report from the National Institute of Animal Science, No. 546, København (1983)
[9] Just, A., W. C. Sauer, S. Bech-Andersen, H. Jørgensen and B. O. Eggum: Z. Tierphysiol., Tierernähr. u. Futtermittelkde **43**, 83 (1980)
[10] Petry, H. and W. Rapp: Z. Tierphysiol., Tierernähr. u. Futtermittelkde **27**, 181 (1970/71)
[11] Poppe, S., Hanna Meier, H. J. Bennke and E. Stöwe: Arch. Tierernähr. **33**, 379 (1983)
[12] Postel, W.: Zuchter, **26**, 211 (1957)
[13] Sauer, W. C., J. J. Kennelly, F. X. Aherne and R. M. Cichoń: Can. J. Anim. Sci. **61**, 793 (1981)
[14] Sauer, W. C., S. C. Stothers and G. D. Phillips: Can. J. Anim. Sci. **57**, 585 (1977)
[15] Saunders, R. M., H. G. Walker and G. O. Kohler: Poultry Sci. **48**, 1497 (1969)
[16] Sodek, L. and C. M. Wilson: J. Agric. Food Chem. **19**, 1144 (1971)
[17] Taverner, M. R., D. M. Curic and C. J. Rayner: Proc. Austral. Soc. Anim. Prod. **14**, 668 (1982)
[18] Taverner, M. R. and D. J. Farrell: Br. J. Nutr. **46**, 173 (1981 a)
[19] Taverner, M. R. and D. J. Farrell: Br. J. Nutr. **46**, 181 (1981 b)
[20] Taverner, M. R., I. D. Hume and D. J. Farrell: Br. J. Nutr. **46**, 159 (1981)
[21] Żebrowska, Teresa: Rocz. Nauk rol. B-95, 117 (1973)

[22] ŻEBROWSKA TERESA, LUCYNA BURACZEWSKA and H. HORACZYŃSKI: Rocz. Nauk rol. B-99, 99 (1978)
[23] ŻEBROWSKA, TERESA, LUCYNA BURACZEWSKA and HANNA ŻEBROWSKA: Proc. VI Intern. Symp. on Amino Acids, Serock 1981, P. S. P., Warszawa 1984, p. 128

A short form of this paper was presented at the 3rd International Seminar on Digestive Physiology in the Pig, Copenhagen, 1985

Received 5 February 1987

Address of authors:

Dr. LUCYNA BURACZEWSKA
Institute of Animal Physiology and Nutrition
05-110 Jabłonna near Warsaw

Dr. E. SCHULZ and HARRIET SCHRÖDER
Institute of Animal Nutrition, FAL
Bundesallee 50
D - 3300 Braunschweig
BRD

Arch. Anim. Nutr., Berlin 37 (1987) 10, 869–880

The National Institute of Animal Science, Denmark
The Royal Veterinary and Agricultural University, Denmark[1]

G. THORBEK, S. HENCKEL, A. CHWALIBOG[1] and B. O. EGGUM

Studies on nitrogen retention in growing pigs

1. Introduction

Nitrogen retention in growing animals is influenced by external and internal factors. The external factors include protein and energy intake, quality of protein supply (essential amino acids) and environmental conditions, while the internal factors include genetical structure (breeds), sex and age of the animal.

From experiments with young pigs on different protein and energy intake it was concluded that in young pigs "nitrogen retention was a function of protein intake, chemical score and energy intake" (MILLER and PAYNE, 1963), while from experiments with pigs over a longer period of growth it was concluded that "there was an upper limit for nitrogen retention depending of the age of the animal" (MØLLGAARD, 1955). These two points of view are to some extent contradictory as discussed in detail by HOCK and PÜSCHNER (1966) and GEBHARDT (1966). However, they might be combined as stressed by KIELANOWSKI (1972) by assuming that young pigs are unable to eat enough feed to secure maximum nitrogen retention and thereby the theory of MILLER and PAYNE (1963) will be valid. In the later stage of growth the animals will reach a level of nitrogen retention on which a further increment of protein and/or energy will have no influence, but the nitrogen retention will be a function of age in accordance with the theory of MØLLGAARD (1955).

In experiments with younger pigs from 20–50 kg live weight nitrogen retention was found to be a linear function of protein intake (GEBHARDT and MÜLLER, 1971), intake of lysine (POPPE and WIESEMÜLLER, 1968) and proportion between energy and protein intake (McCRACKEN et al., 1980), while experiments with pigs over a longer period of growth (20–100 kg) showed curvilinear relations between nitrogen retention and metabolic live weight (THORBEK, 1975) or live weight and live weight gain (JENTSCH and HOFFMANN, 1977).

A parabolic function for nitrogen retention over a longer period of growth seems preferable (MENKE, 1975 and KIRCHGESSNER, 1978) even if it lately has been stated that "nitrogen retention is increasing linearly to a certain level and then being constant independent of age or weight" (WHITTEMORE, 1986).

Protein norms for growing pigs are based on the knowledge about protein retention in relation to external and internal factors and the way in which the retention curves might be described. Different growth models have been applied on measurements of nitrogen retention in growing pigs and thoroughly discussed by PFEIFFER et al. (1984).

The present paper deals with measurements of nitrogen metabolism in growing pigs fed on different feed compound of high or low biological value combined with different energy levels. The data concerning nitrogen retention have been used in statistical analyses for estimation of the shape and level of the nitrogen retention curves.

2. Materials and methods

2.1. General

The experimental material comprised 60 barrows of Danish Landrace and a total of 470 balance periods during the growth period from 20–85 kg live weight (LW). In the first series (Expt A) 48 barrows were allocated to six different feed compounds of high biological value (HBV), while in the second series (Expt B) 12 barrows were measured on feed compounds of HBV or low biological value (LBV) combined with three levels of energy.

2.2. Animals

In order to facilitate a general application of the results obtained twelve different litters with four barrows from each were used in Expt A, while six barrows from two different litters were applied in Expt B. All pigs aquired at a mean age of 65 days and a mean LW of 18 kg were initially adapted, fed on barley + skim milk powder and treated with Piperazin for deworming before they were allocated to the different diets.

Except for one pig in the last period in Expt A the stipulated rations were eaten and no disturbances were observed. In Expt B all pigs on the LBV-compound suddenly at a LW about 45 kg refused to eat and no measurement in the LW-range 45–55 kg were carried out for this group. After an injection of B + E vitamin (Ephynal, La Roche) the appetite was fully restored and no further disturbances occured during the experiment.

2.3. Diets

Six different feed compounds of HBV consisting of barley (BA), maize (MA) or sorghum (SO) combined with skim milk powder (MI) or a protein mixture (PR) of 2/3 soya bean meal + 1/3 meat bone meal were applied in Expt A. The amount of grain was increased from 500–2400 g/d during the experimental time, while the MI or PR-intake increased from 240–350 g/d in the LW-range 20–35 kg and then it was kept constant. The intake of nitrogen (IN) and gross energy (GE) in eight LW-ranges from 20–85 kg for the MI and PR-groups is shown in Table 1 and 2.

The mean intake of nitrogen for the PR-group was 5.4 g/d higher than for the MI-group, the difference being highly significant. The energy intake was identical for the two groups, thereby the energy intake in relation to nitrogen retention was highest for the MI-group.

All twelve pigs in Expt B received a basal diet of wheat + barley + wheat bran, and then six pigs were supplied with a protein mixture of HBV consisting of 2/3 soya bean meal + 1/3 herring meal, while six pigs were given a LBV-protein supply of 2/3 sun-

Table 1

Expt A. Intake of nitrogen (IN, g/d) in feed compounds of barley (BA), maize (MA) or sorghum (SO) supplied with skim milk powder (MI) or protein mixture (PR)

LW range kg	BA, MA or SO supplied with MI n	Mean	SEM	BA, MA or SO supplied with PR n	Mean	SEM	Differences PR – MI g/d
20–25	24	22.6	0.48	24	26.4	0.32	3.8 xxx
25–30	24	28.3	0.48	24	33.4	0.44	5.1 xxx
30–35	24	33.2	0.71	24	39.1	0.68	5.9 xxx
35–45	23	37.4	0.98	24	43.3	0.93	5.9 xxx
45–55	24	42.2	0.96	24	47.7	0.86	5.5 xxx
55–65	24	46.6	1.27	24	52.3	1.21	5.6 xx
65–75	23	50.7	1.53	24	56.2	1.44	5.5 x
75–85	23	54.2	1.61	24	59.7	1.55	5.5 x

xxx : $P<0.001$, xx : $P<0.01$, x : $P<0.05$

Table 2

Expt A. Intake of gross energy (GE) in feed compounds of barley (BA), maize (MA) or sorghum (SO) supplied with skim milk powder (MI) or protein mixture (PR)

LW range kg	BA, MA or SO supplied with MI n	MJ/d	kJ/kg$^{0.75}$	kJ/g IN	BA, MA or SO supplied with PR n	MJ/d	kJ/kg$^{0.75}$	kJ/g IN
20–25	24	13.28	1285	588	24	13.09	1267	496
25–30	24	16.76	1396	592	24	16.54	1377	495
30–35	24	19.92	1463	600	24	19.68	1446	503
35–45	23	24.20	1521	647	24	24.04	1511	555
45–55	24	28.98	1541	687	24	28.73	1528	602
55–65	24	33.62	1559	721	24	33.38	1548	638
65–75	23	38.06	1573	751	24	37.85	1564	673
75–84	23	42.60	1593	786	24	42.46	1587	711

Table 3

Expt B. Intake of nitrogen (IN) and gross energy (GE) in series with protein supply of high (HBV) or low (LBV) biological value on three different fat levels (LF, MF of HF)

LW range kg	IN (HBV + LBV) (LF + MF + HF) n	g/d	GE (HBV + LBV) LF MJ/d	MF MJ/d	HF MJ/d	GE/IN LF kJ/g	MF kJ/g	HF kJ/g
20–25	12	26.4	13.19	14.38	15.58	500	545	590
25–30	12	34.4	17.14	18.52	19.86	498	538	577
30–35	12	38.9	20.41	22.40	24.39	525	576	627
35–45	12	42.4	24.72	27.08	29.37	583	639	693
45–55	6	45.2	28.59	31.79	34.99	633	703	774
55–65	12	48.8	34.10	38.14	42.17	699	782	864
65–75	11	51.0	39.25	44.30	49.16	770	869	964
75–85	12	56.6	43.62	49.46	55.33	779	883	988

flower seed meal + 1/3 meat bone meal. The basal diet without addition of fat (LF) was given to four pigs, while it was supplemented with lard for the remaining eight pigs, being equally divided in two groups. One group received 30–145 g lard/d (MF), while the other group received 60–290 g/d (HF) during the experimental time. The intake of nitrogen was identical on HBV and LBV-compounds and on all fat levels as shown in Table 3. With three different levels of energy intake the relation between energy and nitrogen (GE/IN) was highest for the HF-group (Table 3).

In Expt A and in Expt B (HBV) the intake of lysine and methionine + cystine increased from 10–18 and from 5–12 g/d respectively, while it was decreased with about 30 % for the pigs in Expt B (LBV). All pigs were supplied with minerals and vitamins according to the Danish norms.

2.4. Plan of experiments

The nitrogen metabolism was in both experiments measured individually in eight consecutive balance periods during the growth period in question. Each balance consisted of a preliminary period of seven days followed by a collection period of seven days. For technical reasons two balances in Expt A and one in Expt B were omitted, thereby the total number of balance periods were 381 in Expt A and 89 in Expt B.

The pigs were kept in individual pens in the stable during the preliminary periods and in individual metabolic crates in the collection periods. The temperature was kept at 22 °C in the beginning of the experiments decreasing to 18 °C in the later periods. The standard procedure for balance experiments at the Institute as described by THORBEK (1975) was followed an the data obtained was analyzed statistically in accordance with SNEDECOR (1956).

3. Results

3.1. Variations between pigs concerning nitrogen retention

A rather large difference between the animals capability for nitrogen retention (RN) on identical diets was observed. The magnitude of the greatest individual differences found in Expt A and B is demonstrated in Table 4.

Table 4
Maximal individual differences in nitrogen retention (RN) between pigs on identical diets in Expt A or B

LW range kg	Expt A (BA+MI) RN, g/d			Expt B (HBV, HF) RN, g/d		
	No. 1	No. 3	Diff.	No. 11	No. 12	Diff.
20–25	14.4	12.0	2.4	13.0	12.8	0.2
25–30	16.5	14.4	2.1	16.1	14.9	1.2
30–35	19.4	16.8	2.6	15.0	12.2	2.8
35–45	21,2	17,9	3,3	18.6	16.9	1.7
45–55	22.1	18.6	3.5	19.9	17.8	2.1
55–65	22.3	20.0	2.3	19.8	18.7	1.1
65–75	22.4	19.7	2.7	20.0	18.3	1.7
75–85	21.5	20.3	1.2	19.8	18.0	1.8

In Expt A pig no. 1 and 3, not being littermates, were fed on an identical feed compound of barley + skim milk powder, while in Expt B no. 11 and 12 were littermates on the same HBV-compound with addition of lard (HF). The mean difference was 2.5 g N/d in Expt A and 1.6 g N/d in Expt B, both differences were highly significant ($P < 0.001$).

3.2. Nitrogen metabolism in Expt A

The amount of digested nitrogen (DN) for the MI and PR-groups is given in Table 5 together with the differences between the two groups. The digestibility was higher for the MI-compounds than for the PR-compounds, but with the higher intake of nitrogen for the PR-group (Table 1) this group showed the highest values for DN in all LW-ranges. A t-test showed that the differences, being in the range from 2.1 to 3.4 g N/d, were significant ($P < 0.05$) to highly significant ($P < 0.001$).

Table 5

Expt A. Digested nitrogen (DN, g/d) in feed compounds of barley (BA), maize (MA) or sorghum (SO) supplied with skim milk powder (MI) or protein mixture (PR)

LW range kg	BA, MA or SO supplied with MI			BA, MA or SO supplied with PR			Differences PR – MI g/d
	n	Mean	SEM	n	Mean	SEM	
20–25	24	19.1	0.23	24	21.2	0.16	2.1 xxx
25–30	24	24.1	0.26	24	27.0	0.30	2.9 xxx
30–35	24	28.3	0.34	24	31.7	0.38	3.4 xxx
35–45	23	31.9	0.48	24	35.1	0.49	3.2 xxx
45–55	24	35.6	0.49	24	38.4	0.45	2.8 xxx
55–65	24	39.2	0.52	24	42.1	0.72	2.9 xx
65–75	23	42.4	0.78	24	45.0	0.84	2.6 x
75–85	23	44.6	0.80	24	47.8	0.85	3.2 xx

xxx : $P < 0.001$, xx : $P < 0.01$, x : $P < 0.05$

Table 6

Expt A. Retained nitrogen (RN, g/d) on feed compounds of barley (BA), maize (MA) or sorghum (SO) supplied with skim milk powder (MI) or protein mixture (PR)

LW range kg	BA, MA or SO supplied with MI			BA, MA or SO supplied with PR			Diff. PR – MI g/d	Total. BA, MA or SO supplied with MI or PR		
	n	Mean	SEM	n	Mean	SEM		n	Mean	SEM
20–25	24	11.2	0.20	24	11.6	0.17	0.4 NS	48	11.4	0.14
25–30	24	14.2	0.33	24	14.9	0.25	0.7 NS	48	14.5	0.21
30–35	24	15.9	0.34	24	16.6	0.33	0.7 NS	48	16.3	0.24
35–45	23	16.8	0.45	24	17.7	0.38	0.9 NS	47	17.3	0.30
45–55	24	18.5	0.40	24	19.2	0.47	0.7 NS	48	18.8	0.31
55–65	24	19.6	0.46	24	20.0	0.40	0.4 NS	48	19.8	0.30
65–75	23	19.9	0.48	24	20.4	0.47	0.5 NS	47	20.1	0.33
75–85	23	20.0	0.46	24	20.2	0.35	0.2 NS	47	20.1	0.28

S : $P > 0.05$

The amount of retained nitrogen (RN) increased for both groups from about 11 to 20 g N/d during the growth period as demonstrated in Table 6. In spite of the significant differences in DN no significant differences ($P>0.05$) were found in RN between the MI and PR-group, and the mean values were calculated. The increase of RN in relation to LW was not linear but showed a decreasing rate of increment.

3.3. Nitrogen metabolism in Expt B

The data from Expt B was divided in two groups in accordance with the biological value of the feed compounds applied, as it was found that the nitrogen metabolism was not influenced by the different levels of energy intake. The intake of nitrogen was identical for the two groups (Table 3), but caused by the higher digestibility of the HBV-compound the group on this compound showed the highest values for DN in all LW-ranges, the differences being highly significant ($P<0.01$ or $P<0.001$) as shown in Table 7.

Table 7

Expt B. Digested nitrogen (DN, g/d) in series with protein supply of high (HBV) or low (LBV) biological value on three different fat levels (LF, MF or HF)

LW range kg	HBV (LF+MF+HF) n	Mean	SEM	LBV (LF+MF+HF) n	Mean	SEM	Differences HBV−LBV g/d
20–25	6	21.8	0.31	6	20.2	0.21	1.6 xx
25–30	6	28.5	0.31	6	24.9	0.12	3.6 xxx
30–35	6	32.1	0.26	6	28.5	0.20	3.6 xxx
35–45	6	34.9	0.37	6	32.3	0.35	2.6 xxx
45–55	6	38.3	0.20	–	–	–	–
55–65	6	41.2	0.29	6	38.1	0.42	3.1 xxx
65–75	6	42.2	0.33	5	39.7	0.51	2.5 xx
75–85	6	47.4	0.40	6	44.7	0.70	2.7 xx

xxx: $P<0.001$, xx: $P<0.01$

Table 8

Expt B. Retained nitrogen (RN, g/d) in series with protein supply of high (HBV) or low (LBV) biological value on three different fat levels (LF, MF or HF)

LW range kg	HBV (LF+MF+HF) n	Mean	SEM	LBV (LF+MF+HF) n	Mean	SEM	Differences HBV−LBV g/d
20–25	6	12.5	0.26	6	7.6	0.24	4.9 xxx
25–30	6	14.4	0.41	6	9.9	0.15	4.5 xxx
30–35	6	13.9	0.42	6	11.1	0.19	2.8 xxx
35–45	6	17.3	0.59	6	13.0	0.19	4.3 xxx
45–55	6	17.5	0.67	–	–	–	–
55–65	6	19.1	0.48	6	16.0	0.25	3.1 xxx
65–75	6	18.4	0.46	5	15.5	0.20	2.9 xxx
75–85	6	20.6	0.76	6	17.5	0.47	3.1 xx

xxx: $P<0.001$, xx: $P<0.01$

The amount of retained nitrogen (RN) for both groups is shown in Table 8. In the group on the HBV-compound the RN-values increased from 12.5 to 20.6 g N/d being close to the results obtained in Expt A and with no linearity between RN and LW (cf. Table 6).

The pigs on the LBV-compound showed lower RN-values increasing only from 7.6 to 17.5 g N/d, but similar to the pigs on the HBV-compound the retention was not influenced by the different levels of energy intake. A t-test showed that the differences between the two groups were in the range from 2.8 to 4.9 g N/d being highly significant ($P<0.01$ or $P<0.001$).

3.4. Nitrogen retention curves in Expt A and B

The measurements of nitrogen retention in Expt A and B showed that RN was curvilinear in relation to live weight as well as to metabolic live weight ($kg^{0.75}$). The relation to metabolic live weight for Expt A and for Expt B on HBV or LBV-compound respectively is demonstrated in Fig. 1.

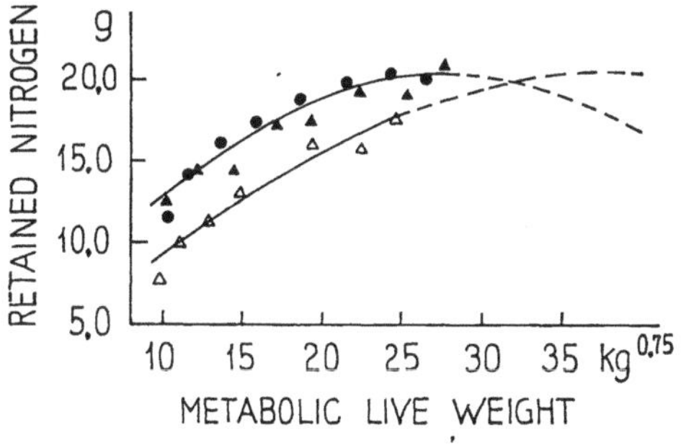

Fig. 1. Nitrogen retention in relation to metabolic live weight in Expt A (●), Expt B, HBV (▲) and Expt B, LBV (△)

By using all individual figures in statistical analyses it was found that a parabolic function of RN on metabolic live weight ($kg^{0.75}$) gave the best fit to the data. The calculations showed that in all regressions the intercept was not significant and for that reason the regression equations were calculated without intercept and the following equations were obtained:

(1) *Expt A* (All compounds)	RN, g/d = 1.48 LW, $kg^{0.75}$ − 0.027 LW, $kg^{1.50}$	
	SE 0.023 0.0011	
	RSD = 1.99 CV = 11.5 % $R^2 = 0.682$ n = 381	
	Maximum = 20.6 g RN/d at 84 kg LW	
(2) *Expt B* (HBV)	RN, g/d = 1.42 LW, $kg^{0.75}$ − 0.025 LW, $kg^{1.50}$	
	SE 0.046 0.0020	
	RSD = 1.47 CV = 8.8 % $R^2 = 0.771$ n = 48	
	Maximum = 20.2 g RN/d at 86 kg LW	
(3) *Expt B* (LBV)	RN, g/d = 1.03 LW, $kg^{0.75}$ − 0.013 LW, $kg^{1.50}$	
	SE 0.035 0.0017	
	RSD = 0.95 CV = 7.4 % $R^2 = 0.944$ n = 41	
	Maximum = 20.4 g RN/d at 133 kg LW	

There was no significant difference ($P<0.01$) between equation (1) and (2) and the common equation was calculated as follows:

$$\text{(4) } \textit{Expt } A+B\ (HBV)\ \text{RN, g/d} = 1.48\ \text{LW, kg}^{0.75} - 0.027\ \text{LW, kg}^{1.50}$$
$$\text{SE} \quad 0.021 \quad 0.0010$$
$$\text{RSD} = 1.95 \quad \text{CV} = 11.3\ \% \quad R^2 = 0.681 \quad n = 429$$
$$\text{Maximum} = 20.5\ \text{g RN/d at 84 kg LW}$$

All regression coefficients were highly significant ($P<0.01$) and the negative coefficients to $kg^{1.50}$ indicate a parabolic form of the regression curves.

4. Discussion

In the present experiments the intake of protein was slightly below the norm given by SCHIEMANN et al. (1971) and by MAFF (1978) in the lower and higher LW-ranges, but the intake of lysine and methionine+cystine on HBV was in accordance with BOLDUAN et al. (1981) and HOFFMANN and WIESEMÜLLER (1981). In order to avoid feed residuals the feed intake was restricted but near ad libitum with energy intake increasing from about 1300 to 1600 GE, kJ/kg$^{0.75}$ in Expt A and in Expt B without addition of fat (LF) and from 1500 to 2100 GE, kJ/kg$^{0.75}$ in Expt B with addition of fat (HF).

The proportion between energy and nitrogen intake increased from 500 to 750 GE, kJ/g IN and from 600 to 1000 GE, kJ/g IN in Expt B on high fat level (HF). The proportion for the younger pigs was in accordance with the optimum proportion found by MCCRACKEN et al. (1980) in experiments with young pigs. In fast growing pigs the increment of energy intake will normally be greater than the increment of nitrogen intake thereby causing an increasing proportion between energy and nitrogen as found in the present experiments. It might be assumed that the intake of protein and essential amino acids and the proportion between energy and nitrogen intake have been sufficient to secure a maximum nitrogen retention for the pigs on feed compounds with a high biological value.

Before discussing the nitrogen retention and the curves obtained it should be stressed, that the experiments indicated that each pig kept its own parameter concerning nitrogen retention during the growth period in question, maintaining a constant difference between individuals. The maximal individual differences were in mean 2.5 and 1.6 g RN/d respectively in Expt A and B (Table 4). This indicates that individual differences in capability of protein formation from the same source of protein intake could vary 10–20 % even for littermates.

In Expt A all pigs on the PR-compounds received more nitrogen than the pigs on the MI-compounds, and the mean difference of 5.4 g IN/d was significant (Table 1). Caused by a loweer digestibility of nitrogen in the protein mixture the mean difference between the two groups was reduced to 2.9 g DN/d, but the difference was still significant (Table 5). In spite of the differences in DN in all LW-ranges no significant differences were found in retained nitrogen (RN) between the two groups (Table 6), and RN increased from 11.4 g RN/d for the younger pigs to 20.1 g RN/d for the older pigs. The rate of increment was not constant in relation to LW but highest for the younger pigs, which indicates a curvilinear function of RN to LW. The standard error of mean (SEM) were in the range 0.14–0.31, corresponding to coefficients of variation ($CV = SD/\bar{x}$) from 8.5 to 11.9 %. The relative great CV-values may be caused mainly be the differences between individuals in their capability for protein formation as discussed earlier.

In Expt B the intake of nitrogen was identical for the pigs on HBV and LBV-compounds, but caused by a higher digestibility of nitrogen in the HBV-compound the DN-values were highest for the pigs on this compound with a mean difference of 2.8 g DN/d being highly significant (Table 7). The nitrogen retention on the HBV-compound increased from 12.5–20.6 g RN/d during the growth period in question, and no influence on the retention was found by increasing the energy intake. On the LBV-compound the RN-values were significantly lower increasing from 7.6–17.5 g RN/d and as for the other group not influenced by the different levels of energy. The CV-values were between 5.1–9.3 % for the pigs on the HBV-compound but somewhat lower between 2.9–7.6 % for the pigs on the LBV-compound. The reason for the lower variation on this compound might be that the genetical differences between the individuals in their capability for protein formation will not be fully unfold on a diet in which the amount of essential amino acids is too low to secure maximum nitrogen retention.

The nitrogen retention measured in Expt B on the HBV-compound was close to the values obtained in Expt A with six different feed compounds of HBV and close to similar experimetns with barrows (Oslage et al., 1966; Bowland et al., 1970; Just (Nielsen), 1970; Gebhardt and Müller, 1971; Wenk, 1973; Böhme et al., 1982). Lower values were obtained in experiments with barrows from 30–130 kg LW (Jentsch and Hoffmann, 1977), which may have been caused by a protein intake being too low to obtain maximum nitrogen retention. Higher RN-values have been observed in experiments with boars (Berschauer et al., 1983) or in experiments with barrows on compensatory growth (Gädeken et al., 1983).

It might be concluded from the present results, that the intake of protein (essential amino acids), energy and energy in relation to nitrogen (i.e. external factors) in Expt A und Expt B (HBV) has been sufficient for the pigs to reach maximum nitrogen retention in the different LW-ranges as no further increment of nitrogen (Expt A) or energy (Expt B) did increase the nitrogen retention. The data was then used to estimate the shape and level of such maximum nitrogen retention curves in relation to LW/age (internal factors). For comparison the curve for the pigs in Expt B on the LBV-compound was estimated as well.

Decreasing increments of nitrogen retention in relation to LW indicate curvilinear functions, but a better fit was obtained by using metabolic live weight ($kg^{0.75}$) as independent variable. RN as a parabolic function of $kg^{0.75}$ was then applied to give regression equations for nitrogen retention in the different series. The equations obtained (1), (2) and (3) showed highly significant negative regression coefficients to the quadratic term ($kg^{1.50}$), which indicate maximum values of RN followed by declining values for older pigs. For a shorter period of growth it is possible to describe RN-curves with linear functions on metabolic live weight or live weight. However, the present results indicate curvlinearity over the growth period from 20–90 kg.

The equations obtained in Expt A (1) and in Expt B (HBV) (2) were not significantly different and a common equation (4) gave a maximum nitrogen retention of 20.5 g/d at a live weight of 84 kg. Thereby demonstrating that as long as the protein and energy supply (external factors) is sufficient an identical parabolic RN-curve will be obtained depending of the internal factors (age, LW and genetical structure).

From Expt B (LBV) the parabolic function (3) gave a maximum of 20.4 g RN/d obtained at a LW of 133 kg. This might indicate that pigs on an insufficient protein supply maintain their growth potential but it will take longer time to reach the maximum.

Summary

Nitrogen retention (RN) was measured in 60 barrows of Danish Landrace and a total of 470 balance periods was carried out during the growth period from 20 to 85 kg live weight. In the first serie (Expt A) six different feed compounds of high biological value (HBV) were fed to 48 barrows, while in the second serie (Expt B) 12 barrows were measured on feed compounds of HBV or low biological value (LBV). Three different levels of gross energy were used in Expt B.

Individual differences of 10–20% in the pigs capability for nitrogen retention were observed.

Nitrogen retention increased from 12 to 21 g N/d on the HBV-compounds and was not influenced by increasing nitrogen or energy intake.

Nitrogen retention was curvilinear in relation to metabolic live weight ($kg^{0.75}$) in both series.

A parabolic function on $kg^{0.75}$ gave the best fit to the data with the following regression equations:

Expt A+B: RN, g/d $= 1.48$ LW, $kg^{0.75} - 0.027$ LW, $kg^{1.50}$
(HBV) Maximum $= 20.5$ g RN/d at 84 kg LW
Expt B: RN, g/d $= 1.03$ LW, $kg^{0.75} - 0.013$ LW, $kg^{1.50}$
(LBV) Maximum $= 20.4$ g RN/d at 133 kg LW

Zusammenfassung

GRETE THORBEK, S. HENCKEL, A. CHWALIBOG und B. EGGUM

Untersuchungen zum Stickstoffansatz bei wachsenden Schweinen

An 60 Börgen der Dänischen Landrasse wurde der Stickstoffansatz (RN) in 470 Bilanzperioden während der Wachstumsperiode von 20 bis 85 kg Lebendmasse gemessen. In der 1. Serie (Versuch A) wurden an 48 Börgen 6 verschiedene Futterkomponenten mit einer hohen biologischen Wertigkeit des Proteins (HBV) verabreicht, während in der 2. Serie (Versuch B) 12 Börge Futterkomponenten einer HBV oder niedrigen biologischen Wertigkeit (LBV) erhielten. Im Versuch B wurden 3 unterschiedliche Niveaus an Bruttoenergie verwendet.

Hinsichtlich der N-Ansatzkapazität wurden 10–20 % individuelle Differenzen beobachtet.

Der N-Ansatz nahm von 12 auf 21 g N/d zu, wenn die HBV-Diäten gefüttert wurden und keine Beeinflussung durch zunehmende N-Einnahme oder Energieeinnahme vorlag.

Der N-Ansatz ließ sich in beiden Versuchsserien in Relation zur metabolischen Körpermasse ($kg^{0,75}$) kurvenförmig darstellen.

Zur metabolischen Körpermasse gab eine parabolische Funktion die beste Angleichung an die entsprechenden Daten mit folgenden Regressionsgleichungen:

Versuche A + B (HBV): RN, g/d = $1{,}48^{0,75}$ kg − 0,027 $kg^{1,50}$
Maximum = 20,5 g RN/d bei 84 kg LM
Versuch B (LBV): RN, g/d = 1,03 $kg^{0,75}$ − 0,013 $kg^{1,50}$
Maximum = 20,4 g RN/d bei 133 kg LM

Резюме

Грете Торбек, С. Хенкель, А. Хвалибог и Б. Эггум

Исследование по отложению азота у растущих свиней

Проводились опыты на 60 боровах породы «*Данский ландграс*», где опредепилось отложение азота (ОА) в 470 балансовых периодах во время ростового периода от 20 до 85 кг живой массы. В первой серии (опыт А) 48 боровов получили 6 различных компонентов корма с высокой биологической ценностью протеина (ВБЦ), а во второй серии (опыт В) 12 боровов получили корма с ВБЦ или с низкой биологической ценностью протеина (НБЦ). В опыте В применялись 3 различных уровня бруттоэнергии.

Наблюдали относительно отложения азота 10–20 % индивидуальные различия.

Отложение азота повышалось от 12 до 21 г азота в сутки, если скармливались диеты с ВБЦ и нет влияния с стороны повышения потребления азота или энергии.

Отложение азота в обоих опытах описывается кривой в отношении с метаболической живой массой ($кг^{0,75}$).

Следующая параболическая функция к метаболической живой массе даёт с помощью следующих уравнений регресси наилучшие данные:

Опыты А + В (ВБЦ): ОА, г/день = 1,48 $кг^{0.75}$ − 0,027 $кг^{1,50}$
Максимум = 20,5 г ОА/день при 84 кг ЖМ
Опыт В (НБЦ): ОА, г/день = 1,03 $кг^{0,75}$ − 0,013 $кг^{1,50}$
Максимум 20,4 г = ОА/день при 133 кг ЖМ

References

[1] Berschauer, F., W. H. Close and D. B. Stephens: Br. J. Nutr. **49**, 271 (1983)

[2] Bolduan, G., L. Hoffmann, K. Keinert and H. Jung: Tierzucht **35**, 124 (1981)

[3] Bowland, J. P., H. Bickel, H. P. Pfirter, C. P. Wenk and A. Schürch: J. Anim. Sci. **31**, 491 (1970)

[4] Böhme, H., D. Gädeken and H. J. Oslage: 9th Symp. on Energy Metabolism. EAAP Publ. **29**, 206 (1982)

[5] Gebhardt, G.: Die Bewertung der Eiweißqualität von Nahrungs- und Futtermitteln mit Hilfe des N-Bilanzversuches. In Vergleichende Ernährungslehre des Menschen und seiner Haustiere. (ed. A. Hock) pp. 323–348. VEB Gustav Fischer Verl. Jena (1966)

[6] Gebhardt, G. and H. Müller: Arch. Tierernähr. **21**, 183 (1971)

[7] GÄDEKEN, D., H. BÖHME and H. J. OSLAGE: Arch. Tierernähr. **33**, 125 (1983)
[8] HOCK, A. and A. PÜSCHNER: Aminosäurestoffwechsel und Nahrungsbedarf. In Vergleichende Ernährungslehre des Menschen und seiner Haustiere. (ed. A. HOCK) pp. 281–321. VEB Gustav Fischer Verl. Jena (1966)
[9] HOFFMANN, L. and W. WIESEMÜLLER: Tierzucht, Berlin, **35**, 222 (1981)
[10] JENTSCH, W. and L. HOFFMANN: Arch. Tierernähr. **27**, 491 (1977)
[11] JUST (NIELSEN), A.: Nat. Inst. Anim. Sci. Denmark. Beretn. **381** (1970)
[12] KIELANOWSKI, J.: Protein requirements of growing animals. In Hdb. Tierernährung. (ed. W. LENKEIT, K. BREIREM & E. CRASEMANN) Bd. II, pp 528–546. Parey Hamburg–Berlin (1972)
[13] KIRCHGESSNER, M.: Tierernährung. DLG Verl. Frankfurt (1978)
[14] MAFF. Ministry of Agriculture, Fisheries and Food. Nutrient Allowances for Pigs. Advisory Paper No. 7 (1978)
[15] MCCRACKEN, K. J., S. M. EDDIE and W. G. STEVENSON: Br. J. Nutr. **43**, 289 (1980)
[16] MENKE, K. H.: Übers. Tierernähr. **3**, 143 (1975)
[17] MILLER, D. S. and P. R. PAYNE: J. Theoret. Biol. **5**, 398 (1963)
[18] MØLLGAARD, H.: Nat. Inst. Anim. Sci. Denmark. Beretn. **282** (1955)
[19] OSLAGE, H. J., H. FLIEGEL, F. E. FARRIES and K. RICHTER: Z. Tierphysiol. Tierernähr. Futtermittelkde. **21**, 50 (1966)
[20] PFEIFFER, H., G. von LENGERKEN and G. GEBHARDT: Wachstum und Schlachtkörperqualität bei landwirtschaftlichen Nutztieren – Schweine. VEB Dt. Landwirtschaftsverl. Berlin (1984)
[21] POPPE, S. and W. WIESEMÜLLER: Arch. Tierernähr. **18**, 392 (1968)
[22] SCHIEMANN, R., K. NEHRING, L. HOFFMANN, W. JENTSCH and A. CHUDY: Energetische Futterbewertung und Energienormen. VEB Landwirtschaftsverl. Berlin (1971)
[23] SNEDECOR, G. W.: Statistical Methods Applied to Expriments in Agriculture and Biology. The Iowa State College Press. (1956)
[24] THORBEK, G.: Nat. Inst. Anim. Sci. Denmark. Beretn. **424** (1975)
[25] WENK, C.: Einfluß verschieden hoher Zufuhr von Futterenergie und Futterprotein auf den Gesamtstoffwechsel, die Mastleistung und die Schlachtkörperzusammensetzung wachsender Schweine. Diss. E. T. H., aku-Fotodruck, Zürich (1973)
[26] WHITTEMORE, C. T.: Proc. Nutr. Soc. **45**, 111 (1986)

Received 11 March 1987

Address of authors:

Dr. A. CHWALIBOG
Department of Animal Nutrition
The Royal Veterinary and Agricultural University
Bülowsvej 13, Frederiksberg C
DK - 1870
Denmark

Arch. Anim. Nutr., Berlin 37 (1987) 10, 881–894

Estación Experimental del Zaidín (C.S.I.C.), Granada, Spain

J. F. AGUILERA and C. PRIETO

Effect of protein quality on energy requirements for maintenance in growing rats

1. Introduction

Nitrogen retention depends to a great extent on amino acid supply and therefore on the quantity and/or the quality (biological value) of protein. Although contradictory results have been published, it has become generally accepted that increases in body protein retention are associated with higher rates of both protein synthesis and protein breakdown (GOLDEN et al., 1977; REEDS et al., 1980; REEDS et al., 1981). It has also been reported that rats offered diets of low protein content have higher metabolizable energy for maintenance (ME_m) associated with lower efficiencies of utilization of energy (BLACK et al., 1955; MILLER and PAYNE, 1962; MCCRACKEN, 1968a; ROTHWELL et al., 1983; LUNN and AUSTIN, 1983) than rats fed on optimal levels of dietary protein. Moreover the utilization of dietary energy by young lambs (WALKER and NORTON, 1971) and growing pigs (HOLMES et al., 1979; CLOSE and BERSCHAUER, 1980) can also be influenced by the concentration of protein in the diet. However, no information has been found in the literature on the extent to which ME_m and the relative cost of protein and fat deposition are modified by the protein quality of the diet. In a previous work (PRIETO and AGUILERA, 1986) rats given several sources of dietary protein which differ widely in their biological value showed marked differences in nitrogen retention and subsequently in level of production and relative rate of protein: fat deposition. The aim of the present work was to get additional information on this subject and to determine whether or not variations in ME_m attributable to dietary protein quality (per se or through induced variations in body composition, or both) can be detected by the classical models of partitioning ME.

2. Materials and methods

2.1. Animals and diets

Forty male Wistar rats were weaned at 21 d and then grouped into six weight blocks (initial weight 45–50 g). Each group was allocated to one of 6 dietary treatments for four weeks (weeks I to IV). Then over weeks V and VI the rats were fed on the same diets but restricted to 60 % of the voluntary feed intake. Six isocaloric and isonitrogenous semisynthetic diets (PRIETO and AGUILERA, 1986) based on soya bean meal (diet SBM) or ground lupin (Lupinus albus var. multolupa) seed (diet LS) alone or autoclaved (A) or not at 120 °C and supplemented with DL-methionine (diets ALS_m or LS_m, respectively) or with DL-methionine + L-Lysine (diets ALS_{m+l} or LS_{m+l}) were prepared (Table 1). In a parallel experiment an additional group of eight rats was given ad libitum the diet SBM and, after a period of 4 weeks, the animals were fasted for 72 h and then fed on the previous diet at a level of intake slightly below maintenance stipulated on basis of body weight.

Table 1

Composition of semisynthetic diets based on soya bean meal (diet SBM) or lupin seed meal (diet LS)

Ingredients (g kg^{-1})	SBM	LS*
Lupin seed meal	–	291
Soya bean meal	243	–
Maize oil	40	26
Cellulose	31	12
Sucrose	314	302
Maize starch	325	322
Vitamin mixture	10	10
Mineral mixture	35	35
Choline chloride	2	2
Chemical composition		
Total N (DM, %)	1.51 – 1.57	
Gross energy (MJ kg^{-1} DM)	18.1 –19.3	
Metabolizable energy (MJ kg^{-1} DM)	15.4 –17.0	
Dry matter (DM, %)	93.1 –94.3	

* Some diets based on ground lupin seed autoclaved or not at 120 °C were supplemented with 2 g DL-methionine kg^{-1} (diets ALS_m or LS_m, respectively) or with 2 g DL-methionine + 1 g L-lysine. kg^{-1} (diets ALS_{m+l} or LS_{m+l}) at the expense of maize starch.

2.2. Experimental procedure

All animals were kept in individual metabolic crates placed in an environmentally controlled room at 23 °C and 70 % RH and had been offered their respective diets for at least one week before the respiration measurements began. Energy metabolism was measured using an open circuit respiration facility described elsewhere (AGUILERA and PRIETO, 1985). As only two chambers were available, 24 h respiration measurements were performed, after a 24 h adaptation period, on groups of 2 rats each (two individual cages inside each of the two chambers) over weeks I to VI. Gas exchange measurements were also carried out on the additional group of eight rats over weeks II to VII. Over the 24 h respiration experiment feed intakes and urinary and faecal losses were accurately controlled. In order to calculate the individual energy metabolism, the measured amounts of O_2 consumption and CO_2 production were divided by two and the individual feed intakes for the period taken into account. Total heat production was calculated according to the equation proposed by BROUWER (1965). The gross energy of feeds and freeze-dried faeces and urine was measured in an adiabatic bomb calorimeter. Total N was determined in feeds, urine and faeces by the micro-

Table 2

Experimental design of the gas exchange measurements

Diet	Feeding level	No of rats	Period of age (weeks)
SBM	Ad libitum	4	II, III, IV
	Restricted*	4	V, VI
LS	Ad libitum	4	II, III, IV
	Restricted*	4	V, VI
LS_m	Ad libitum	8	I, II, III, IV
	Restricted*	8	V, VI
ALS_m	Ad libitum	8	I, II, III, IV
	Restricted*	8	V, VI
LS_{m+l}	Ad libitum	8	I, II, III, IV
	Restricted*	8	V, VI
ALS_{m+l}	Ad libitum	8	I, II, III, IV
	Restricted	8	V, VI
SBM	Fasting	8	IV, VI
	Restricted+	8	II, III, VII

* 60 % ad libitum (above maintenance)
+ Below maintenance

Kjeldahl procedure. The experimental design appears in Table 2. A more detailed desoription of methodology has been published elsewhere (PRIETO and AGUILERA, 1986; AGUILERA et al., 1986).

Regression analysis were used throughout with data being pooled whenever appropriate.

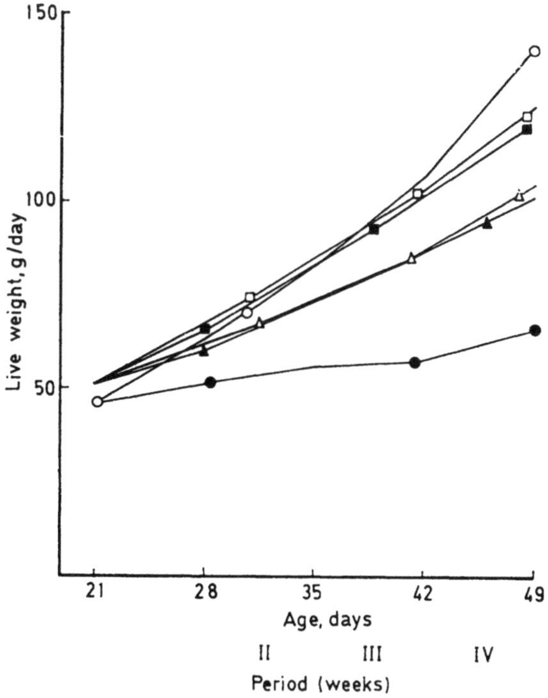

Fig. 1. Live weight in relation to age of rats given ad lib low-protein diets based on soya bean meal (○——○) and lupin seed meal alone (●——●) or autoclaved or not and supplemented with DL-methionine (△——△ or ■——■) or DL-methionine + L-lysine (▲——▲ or □——□).

3. Results

The diets had been formulated to contain restricted amounts of protein in order to provide the adequate experimental conditions to determine the biological value and, consequently, this fact had an effect on growth rate and body composition. Live weight of rats over the 4-week ad libitum feeding period appears in Figure 1. Different levels of production were obtained with the experimental diets (PRIETO and AGUILERA, 1986). Live weight gain (3.43, 0.76, 2.57, 1.95, 2.70 and 1.85 g d^{-1}) was in agreement with the biological value of the dietary protein (60.1, 39.2, 49.9, 45.8, 45.1 and 47.3) for diets SBM, LS, LS_m, ALS_m, LS_{m+l} and ALS_{m+l}, respectively). Mean values of RE and

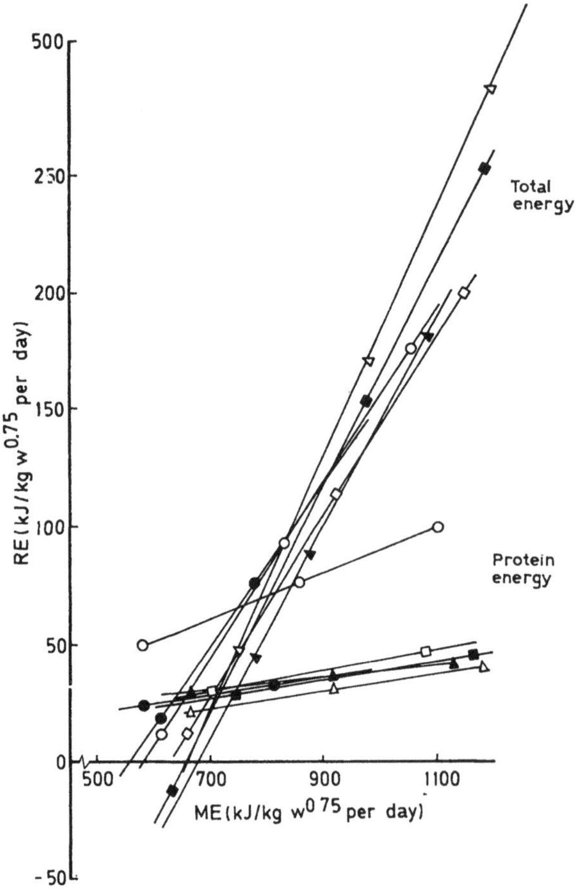

Fig. 2. Energy retained (RE) in rats given low-protein diets at two feeding levels (restricted and ad libitum) based on soya bean meal (○—○—○) and lupin seed meal alone (●—●—●) or autoclaved or not and supplemented with DL-methionine (△—△—△ or ■—■—■ respectively), or DL-methionine + L-lysine (▲—▲—▲ or □—□—□).

energy retained as protein (REP) over weeks I to IV (ad libitum feeding period) were 45.5 and 21.6; 17.0 and 4.9; 43.5 and 7.0; 41.0 and 5.4; 32.7 and 7.8; 28.9 and 5.9 kJ day^{-1}, for diets SBM, LS, LS_m, ALS_m, LS_{m+l} and ALS_{m+l}, respectively. The low protein availability not only affected RE but also the relative rate of energy retained as fat: energy retained as protein, which was high in most groups. The effect of feeding level on energy retention is shown in Figure 2. It should be noticed that when metabolizable energy intake (ME_i) was restricted to 60 % of ad libitum intake, positive nitrogen balances were concomitant of body fat mobilization.

Table 3

Estimates of energy requirements of rats fed on diets of different protein quality at two fixed levels of ME intake

Diet	Levels of ME_i	Linear regression equations	n	RSD	r	ME_m ($kJ/kgW^{0.75}$)*
SBM	Above maintenance RE ($kJ/kgW^{0.75}$)	$= -206 + 0.366$ ME ($kJ/kgW^{0.75}$) SE - (± 10) (± 0.04)	10	33.18	0.965	564
LS	„ „ RE	$= -237 + 0.382$ ME (± 10) (± 0.05)	10	33.14	0.937	621
LS_m	„ „ RE	$= -360 + 0.599$ ME (± 14) (± 0.04)	12	49.87	0.975	602
ALS_m	„ „ RE	$= -357 + 0.599$ ME (± 20) (± 0.06)	12	70.50	0.950	596
LS_{m+1}	„ „ RE	$= -285 + 0.496$ ME (± 16) (± 0.05)	12	53.97	0.955	574
ALS_{m+1}	„ „ RE	$= -325 + 0.545$ ME (± 18) (± 0.06)	12	61.09	0.943	596
Pooled	„ „ RE	$= -327 + 0.546$ ME (± 15) (± 0.04)	68	63.35	0.949	599
SBM	Below maintenance RE	$= -485 + 0.811$ ME (± 11) (± 0.05)	11	35.77	0.986	598

* Value for ME_i when RE = 0

Measurements of energy balance of rats given the different experimental diets at the two feeding levels considered (ad libitum and 60 % ad lib or restricted) have been used to predict the energy intake at zero energy retention, using a linear regression of RE on ME_i:

$$(1) \qquad RE/W^{0.75} = -a + b \times ME_i/W^{0.75}$$

where RE represents the total energy retention ($RE = ME_i$ – total heat production, kJ/kg body weight$^{0.75}$ per d) and ME_i the intake of metabolizable energy. The equation predicts ME for maintenance (ME_m) as the intercept on the x-axis and also provides an estimate of the efficiency of utilization of ME above maintenance. In order to justify the further statistical analysis and estimate the standard deviation of the intercept (ME_m), ME_i has also been regressed on RE. The above equation has also been used to estimate ME_m from measurements on rats fasted or fed on diet SBM at a sub-maintenance level. In this case, b represents the efficiency of utilization of ME for maintenance. Table 3 and Figure 3 summarize the solution to equation (1).

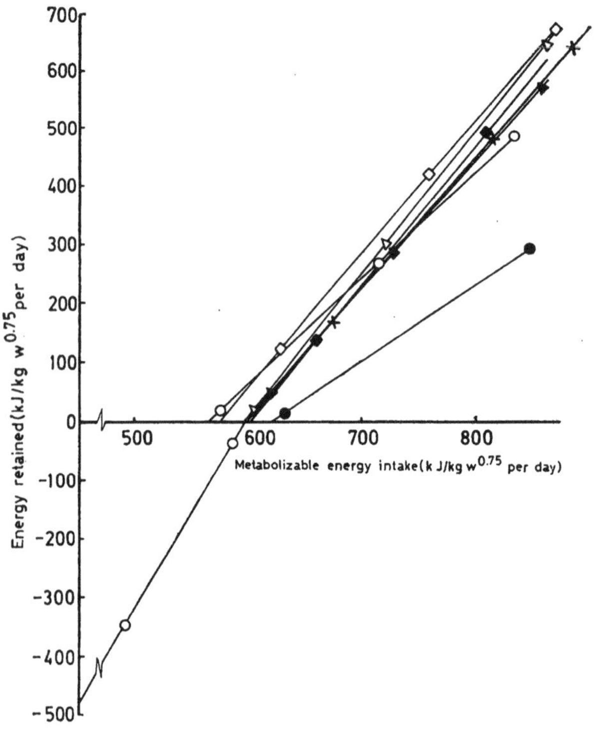

Fig. 3. Effect on the estimates of energy requirements for maintenance in rats of low-protein diets based on soya bean meal (○——○) and lupin seed meal, alone (●——●) or autoclaved or not and supplemented with DL-methionine (△——△ or ■——■ respectively) or DL-methionine + L-lysine (▲——▲ or □——□), pooled data (×——×).

The efficiencies of utilization of ME for production ranged from 36.6 to 59.9 %, the differences being only significant between diet SBM and diets LS_m ($P < 0.001$), ALS_m ($P < 0.01$), LS_{m+l} ($P < 0.05$) and ALS_{m+l} ($P < 0.05$), and between diet LS and diets LS_m ($P < 0.01$) and ALS_m ($P < 0.05$). The estimates for ME_m ranged from 564 to 621 kJ/kgW$^{0.75}$. When regressing ME_i on RE (Table 4), no significant differences between diets were observed. Consequently, further equations for pooled data were also calculated (Tables 3 and 4). An overall value for ME_m of 599 kJ/kgW$^{0.75}$ and an effi-

Table 4
Range of the ME_m estimates for the experimental diets

Diet	Levels of ME_i	Linear regression equations	n	RSD	r	Range of ME_m estimates ($kJ/kgW^{0.75}$)
SBM	Above maintenance ME_i	$=584+2.55$ RE ($kJ/kgW^{0.75}$) SE (± 28) (± 0.25)	10	87.57	0.965	520–648
LS	,, ,, ME_i	$=636+2.30$ RE (± 26) (± 0.31)	10	81.34	0.937	577–696
LS_m	,, ,, ME_i	$=628+1.59$ RE (± 23) (± 0.11)	12	81.17	0.975	576–680
ALS_m	,, ,, ME_i	$=653+1.51$ RE (± 32) (± 0.16)	12	111.93	0.950	581–725
LS_{m+1}	,, ,, ME_i	$=622+1.84$ RE (± 30) (± 0.18)	12	104.05	0.955	555–689
ALS_{m+1}	,, ,, ME_i	$=650+1.63$ RE (± 30) (± 0.18)	12	105.77	0.943	582–718
Pooled	,, ,, ME_i	$=642+1.65$ RE (± 27) (± 0.14)	68	110.80	0.949	615–668
SBM	Below maintenance ME_i	$=589+1.20$ RE (± 13) (± 0.07)	11	43.49	0.986	559–618

ciency on energy utilization for production of 54.6 % were obtained (Table 3). When measuring fasting heat production, the respiratory quotient (RQ) was on average 0.69, indicating complete fat oxidation. From energy balance measurements at fasting and below maintenance levels an estimate for ME_m of 598 kJ/kg$W^{0.75}$, which was not significantly different from those calculated above maintenance, and an efficiency of utilization of ME for maintenance (K_m) of 81.1 % were obtained.

4. Discussion

The present estimates for ME_m are in the range of values reported in the literature (Table 5) and close to those obtained in growing rats given low-protein diets, which are higher than values given for rats fed on optimal levels of protein. It has been shown that low-protein diets affect the composition of tissue gain and may be associated with dietary-induced thermogenesis (ROTHWELL et al., 1983; LUNN and AUSTIN, 1983; COYER et al., 1985). It has also been reported that these diets gave slower growth and also decreased the efficiency of energy retention (MCCRACKEN, 1968a). In addition, CAMPBELL and DUNKIN (1983) obtained increased ME_m and lower efficiency of energy utilization in baby pigs fed on a protein-deficient diet in comparison with a protein-adequate diet. On the contrary, MCCRACKEN and MCALLISTER (1984) in young pigs failed to demonstrate significant changes in estimates for ME_m induced by dietary protein content.

Our results indicate that there are no significant differences in ME_m attributable to variations in protein quality of diets. However it should be pointed out that estimates for ME_m calculated following the conventional way of regressing RE/kg$W^{0.75}$ on ME_i/kg$W^{0.75}$ should be regarded with caution as, among other assumptions, it is supposed that the proportion between energy retained as protein (RPE) and fat (RFE) is constant on high and low feeding levels, a fact which cannot be fulfilled in feeding experiments (HENCKEL, 1976). In this respect, in the present work large differences in the REF : REP relationship were found between restricted and ad libitum feeding levels. The mean value for ME_m of 599 kJ/kg$W^{0.75}$ per d for pooled data is very close to that obtained from measurements at fasting and below maintenance level (598 kJ/kg$W^{0.75}$ per d), which may be an index of the validity of our results. On the other hand, the value of efficiency of energy utilization for maintenance obtained (K_m = 0.811) is in agreement with the theoretical biochemical efficiency.

Our overall value for the apparent efficiency of dietary ME utilization above maintenance of 0.55 (Table 3) falls in line with several reported values for rats in their thermoneutral zone. The slightly lower value for diet SBM is to be expected because of the inherently lower biochemical efficieny of translocation of dietary protein into tissue protein. This might be due to the extra costs associated with protein deposition.

Estimates of ME_m based on measurements of fasting metabolism are usully considered unsatisfactory because they are determined for a physiological state which is remote for normal production as during fasting animals are largely sustained by oxidation of body fat and are suffering from a gross energy deficiency. The question whether estimation of ME_m on low feeding level can be applied to fed animals is still a matter of dispute. EGGUM and CHWALIBOG (1983) found that fed rats seem to have

Table 5

Estimates of energy requirements for maintenance (ME_m, kJ/d per kg body weight$^{0.75}$) in growing rats

Source	Body wt (g)	Crude protein of diet (%)	ME_m	Method of estimation for ME_m
McCracken (1968a)	55– 75	5.0	605	Calculated[1]
McCracken (1968b)	55– 75	5.0–20.0	471–518	Calculated[1]
Vermorel & Keller (1969)	133	15.0	554	RE vs ME_i
McCracken (1975)	50– 70	5.0–10.0	433–461	Direct
Deb et al. (1976)	142–254	22.2	546	RE vs ME_i
Eggum et al. (1982)	80–280	13.0–13.3	549–469	ME_i vs RE
Hoffmann et al. (1982)	65–180	10.0–40.0	437	Direct
	65–180	10.0–40.0	423	Multiple regression
McCracken & Barr (1983)	90	Stock and varied diet	634–692	RE vs ME_i[2]
Lunn & Austin (1983)	100–115	3.0	586	Assumed
Coyer et al. (1985)	104	22.0– 9.0	562–564	ME_i vs RE
Present paper	45–145	10.0	598	RE vs ME_i[3]
	45–145	10.0	599	RE vs ME_i[4]
	45–145	10.0	647	Multiple regression

1 Assuming 31.4 kJ/g protein formed and 66.5 kJ/g fat formed
2 Using a common intercept of -0.45 MJ/kgW$^{0.75}$
3 Below maintenance
4 Above maintenance

a higher ME_m requirements than starved rats. THORBEK et al. (1984) reported that ME_m estimates from fed pigs was up to 20 % higher than from starved pigs. On the contrary, HOFFMAN et al. (1982) in studies with growing rats and broilers could not measure any differences in ME_m values obtained on low feeding levels versus high feeding levels. Our results are in this line, as no differences have been found between the two mentioned approaches (below and above maintenance) for estimating ME requirements.

As in the present experiment no significant differences in ME_m were found among diets, a multiple regression equation (KIELANOWSKI, 1965) on pooled data was used with ME intake as the dependent variable and energy retained as protein (REP) and fat (REF) as independent variables. REP and REF were calculated from experimental results assuming 149.1 kJ/g N and 39.7 kJ/g fat (REF = total energy retention-REP). The equation was:

$$\text{ME (kJ/kgW}^{0.75}) = 647 + 4.55\ \text{REP} + 1.14\ \text{REF}. \quad r = 0.865$$
$$\text{SE } (\pm 12)\ (\pm 0.88)\quad (\pm 0.10) \qquad n = 68$$

The reciprocals of the coefficients of REP and REF represent estimates of efficiency of energy utilization for protein and fat deposition ($K_p = 0.22$ and $K_f = 0.88$, respectively), while the intercept term is an estimate for ME_m (647 kJ/kgW$^{0.75}$ per d). This value differs by around 8 % compared with that obtained when applying the simple regression model (599 kJ/kgW$^{0.75}$ per d). Some of the discrepancies found in ME_m between the two approaches can be explained by the evidence (ROUX et al., 1982) that the multiple regression model proposed by KIELANOWSKI (1965) does not provide reliable data on the energetio efficiency of protein and fat deposition, as the suposedly independent variables in this equation (REP and REF) are in fact correlated. CAMPBELL and DUNKIN (1983) and CLOSE et al. (1983) when comparing protein-adequate with protein-deficient diets have reported that high estimates of K_f are associated with low estimates of K_p, in agreement with our results. It should be noticed that the experimental diets were formulated to contain low levels of protein from moderate to low biological value and this fact must have severely limited the amino acid availability. On the other hand, it is known that the biological quality of dietary protein has an influence upon the rate of N retention. In growing pigs (REEDS et al., 1980) and children (GOLDEN et al., 1977) increases in N retention have been associated with higher rates of both protein synthesis and protein breakdown in the whole body. Thus it should not be descarded the hypothesis that changes in these rates through alterations in the BV of dietary protein may influence the energetic costs of net protein deposition. Unfortunately, the experimental design has proved to be unable to provide information on the effect of dietary protein quality on K_p and K_f. The data presented here were limited and some variances were high, so inconsistent results were found when applying multiple regression equations to individual treatments.

In conclusion, no variations in ME_m requirements in growing rats attributable to either dietary protein quality or statistical method of estimation have been found. Nevertheless, these results should be taken with caution because of limitations inherent of statistical models of partitioning ME, which are unable to reflect the physiological and biochemical processes within the animal.

Summary

Forty 3-week old male Wistar rats (initial weight 45–50 g) were used. After weaning they were fed ad libitum for four weeks (I to IV) on 6 isocaloric and isonitrogenous semisynthetic diets based on soya bean meal (diet SBM) or on ground lupin seed (diet LS) alone or autoclaved (A) or not at 120 °C and supplemented with DL-methionine (diets ALS_m or LS_m, respectively) or with DL-methionine + L-lysine (diets ALS_{m+l} or LS_{m+l}). The diets differ in their protein quality and were formulated in order to provide the adequate experimental conditions to determine the biological value (10 % crude protein). Then over the fifth and sixth weeks (V and VI) the rats were fed on the same diets but restricted to 60 % of the voluntary feed intake. In a parallel experiment, a group of eight rats previously fed ad libitum on diet SBM for four weeks was fasted for 72 h and then fed on the same diet at a level of intake slightly below maintenance. After a 24 h adaptation period, irrespective of the level of intake and type of diet, a series of 24 h gas-exchanges measurements were carried out in open-circuit respiration chambers.

Measurements of energy balance were used to calculate ME for maintenance (ME_m) and the efficiency of utilization of ME, using a linear regression of energy retention (RE) on ME. The estimates for ME_m derived from energy balances of rats fed above maintenance ranged from 564 to 621 kJ/kgW$^{0.75}$ per d. No significant differences between diets were observed. From pooled data ME_m was found to be 599 kJ/kgW$^{0.75}$ per d, a value not significantly different from that calculated from measurements at fasting and below maintenance levels (598 kJ/kgW$^{0.75}$ per d). The efficiency of utilization of ME for maintenance was 81.1 % and the efficiencies of utilization of ME for RE ranged from 36.6 to 59.9 %.

It is concluded that no variations in ME_m requirements in growing rats attributable to variations in dietary protein quality have been found. Nevertheless, these results should be taken with caution because of limitations inherent of statistical modelling approaches of partitioning ME.

Zusammenfassung

J. F. AGUILERA und C. PRIETO

Der Effekt der Proteinqualität auf den Energiebedarf für die Erhaltung bei wachsenden Ratten

Vierzig 3 Wochen alte männliche Wistar-Ratten (Anfangsmasse 45–50 g) wurden verwendet.

Nach der Entwöhnung wurden sie 4 Wochen (I bis IV) mit 6 semisynthetischen Diäten (mit gleichem Energie- und Stickstoffgehalt) ad libitum gefüttert. Die Diäten bestanden aus Sojaextraktionsschrot (Diät SBM), Lupinensamenschrot (Diät LS), autoklaviert (A) bei 120 °C oder nicht autoklaviert, mit Zusätzen von DL-Methionin (Diät ALS_m, beziehungsweise LS_m) oder von DL-Methionin + L-Lysin (Diät ALS_{m+l} oder LS_{m+l}). Die Diäten unterschieden sich in ihrer Proteinqualität und wurden so zusammengesetzt, um die richtigen Bedingungen für die Bestimmung der biologischen Wertigkeit (10 % Rohprotein) zu erreichen. Nach der fünften und sechsten Woche

(V und VI) wurde die Futtergabe auf 60 % des ad libitum aufgenommenen Futters begrenzt. In einem parallelen Versuch erhielt eine Gruppe von 8 Ratten, die vorher für 4 Wochen mit der Diät SBM ad libitum gefüttert worden war, während 72 h keine Futtergabe, danach erhielt sie Futtergaben der gleichen Diät, die knapp unter dem Erhaltungsbedarf lagen.

Nach einer Adaptionszeit von 24 Stunden wurden, unabhängig von der Aufnahmemenge und Art der Diät, über 24 h, in einer Respirationsanlage nach dem „offenen Prinzip", Messungen des Gaswechsels vorgenommen.

Die Messungen zur Energiebilanz wurden benutzt, um die umsetzbare Energie (ME) für den Erhaltungsbedarf (ME_m) und den Wirkungsgrad der ME über eine lineare Regression von retinierter Energiemenge (RE) zur aufgenommenen ME zu berechnen.

Berechnungen der ME_m, ausgehend von der Energiebilanz von Ratten mit Rationen über dem Erhaltungsbedarf, reichten von 564 bis 621 $kJ/kg^{0,75} \cdot d$.

Es wurden keine signifikanten Unterschiede zwischen den Diäten beobachtet. Ausgehend von allen vorliegenden Ergebnissen betrug die ME_m 599 $kJ/kg^{0,75}$ pro Tag, ein Wert, der nicht signifikant von dem Wert aus Messungen während der Periode ohne Futtergabe und unterhalb des Erhaltungsbedarfs (598 $kJ/kg^{0,75}$), abweicht. Der Nutzungsgrad der ME für den Erhaltungsbedarf betrug 81,1 % und der Nutzungsgrad der ME für die retinierte Energie lag zwischen 36,6 % and 59,9 %.

Eine Änderung des ME-Bedarfs bei wachsenden Ratten in Abhängigkeit von der Proteinqualität konnte nicht ermittelt werden. Diese Ergebnisse sollten, aufgrund der begrenzten Aussagefähigkeit von statistischen Modellen, nicht überbewertet werden.

Резюме

И. Ф. Агуилера и Ц. Приего

Эффект качества протеина на потребность для поддержания жизни у растущих крыс

40 ♂ крыс породы «Вистар» в возрасте 3 недель с 45–50 г живой массы служили опытом.

После отьёма они ввлою получили в течение 4 недель (I–IV) 6 полусинтетические диеты с равным содержанием энергии и протеина. Диеты состояли из соевого шрота (диета 5 BM), шрот из люпинных семён (диета LS), автоклавированная (A) при 120 °C или неавтоклавированная, с добавками DL-метионина (диета ALS_m или LS_m) или DL-метионина + L-лизина (диета ALS_{m+1} или LS_{m+1}).

Диеты различились относительно их качества протеина и смешались (10 % сырого протеина) таким образом, чтобы получить правильные условия для определения биологической ценности протеина. Потребление кормов ограничивалось после 5-ой и 6-ой недель до 60 % потребления ввлою. В параллельном опыте группа с 8 крысами скармливалась ввлою во время 4 недель диетой SBM, а затем не получила никакого корма за 72 час, а после этого натощака кормили крысам с самой диетой только немного ниже потребности для поддерживания жизни. После 24 часов адаптации определился в газовой обмен в респирационной системе по «открыкрытому принципу» и независимо от вида диеты и её количества потребления.

Измерения баланса энергии служили вычислением с помощью линейной регрессии обменной энергии (ME) для потребности для поддерживания жизни (ME_m) и для эффективности ME от отложенного (ретинированного) количества энергии (RE) к потребленной ME.

Вычисления ME_m исходя от баланса энергии у крыс, получавших рационы выше потребности для поддерживания жизни, колебались от 564 до 621 кДж/кг^{0,75} · d. Обнаружили, что нет достоверных разлигий между диетами. Исходя от всех полученных результатов, можно выводить, что ME_m в сутки = 599 кДж/кг^{0,75}, что только недостоверно различается от данных из периодов без кормов и ниже потребности для поддержания жизни (598 кДж/кг$^{0.75}$). Степень использования ME для поддержания жизни составила 81,1 %, а для ретинированной энергии она находилась между 36,6 и 59,9 %. Не было изменения потребности ME у растущих крыс в зависимости от качества протеина. Следует эти результати в дальнейшем уточнить, потому что выоды из статистической модели ограничы.

References

[1] Aguilera. J. F. and C. Prieto: Arch. Tierernähr. **35**, 781 (1985)
[2] Aguilera, J. F., C. Prieto, J. Fonolla and F. Gil: Anim. Feed Sci. Technol. **15**, 33 (1986)
[3] Black, A., K. H. Maddy and R. W. Swift: J. Nutr. **42**, 415 (1955)
[4] Brouwer, E.: Report of Sub-Committee on Constants and Factors. Proc. 3rd Symp. on Energy Metabolism, Troon, EAAP Publ. No. **11**, 441 (1965)
[5] Campbell. R. G. and C. Dunkin: Br. J. Nutr. **49**, 221 (1983)
[6] Close, W. H. and F. Berschauer: Proc. Nutr. Soc. **40**, 33A (1980)
[7] Close, W. H., F. Berschauer and R. P. Heavens: Br. J. Nutr. **49**, 255 (1983)
[8] Coyer, P., J. P. W. Rivers and D. J. Millward: Proc. Nutr. Soc. **44**, 131A (1985)
[9] Deb, S., R. J. Martin and T. V. Hershberger: J. Nutr. **106**, 191 (1976)
[10] Eggum, B. O., G. Thorbek, R. M. Beames, A. Chwalibog and S. Henckel: Br. J. Nutr. **48**, 161 (1982)
[11] Eggum, B. O. and A. Chwalibog: Z. Tierphysiol. Tierernähr. u. Futtermittelkde. **49**, 104 (1983)
[12] Golden, M. H. N., J. C. Waterlow and D. Picou: Am. J. Clin. Nutr. **30**, 1345 (1977)
[13] Henckel, S.: Statistical methods for estimation of maintenance requirements and efficiencies in animal production during growth. Proc. 7th Symp. on Energy Metabolism, Vichy, EAAP Publ. No. **19**, 145 (1976)
[14] Hoffman, L., M. Klein and R. Schiemann: Arch. Tierernähr. **32**, 165 (1982)
[15] Holmes, C. W., R. Christensen, J. R. Carr and G. Pearson: Some aspects of the energy metabolism of growing pigs fed on diets containing different concentration of protein. Proc. 8th Symp. on Energy Metabolism, Cambridge, EAAP Publ. No. **26**, 97 (1979)
[16] Kielanowski, J.: Estimates of the energy cost of protein deposition in growing animals. Proc. 3rd Symp. on Energy Metabolism, Troon, EAAP Publ. No. **11**, 13 (1965)
[17] Lunn, P. G. and S. Austin: Br. J. Nutr. **49**, 9 (1983)
[18] McCracken, K. J.: Proc. Nutr. Soc. **27**, 40A (1968a)
[19] McCracken, K. J.: Proc. Nutr. Soc. **27**, 41A (1968b)
[20] McCracken, K. J.: Br. J. Nutr. **33**, 277 (1975)
[21] McCracken, K. J. and H. G. Barr: Proc. Nutr. Soc. **42**, 3A (1983)
[22] McCracken, K. J. and A. McAllister: Br. J. Nutr. **51**, 225 (1984)
[23] Miller, D. S. and P. R. Payne: J. Nutr. **78**, 255 (1962)

[24] PRIETO, C. and J. F. AGUILERA: J. Anim. Physiol. a Anim. Nutr. **55**, 239 (1986)
[25] REEDS, P. J., A. CADENHEAD, M. F. FULLER, G. E. LOBLEY and J. D. McDONALD: Br. J. Nutr. **43**, 445 (1980)
[26] REEDS, P. J., M. F. FULLER, A. CADENHEAD, G. E. LOBLEY and J. D. McDONALD: Br. J. Nutr. **45**, 539 (1981)
[27] ROTHWELL, N. J., M. J. STOCK and R. S. TYZBIR: Met. Clin. Exp. **32**, 257 (1983)
[28] ROUX, C. Z., H. S. HOFMEYR and E. JORDAAN: The problem of multicollinearity in the estimation of partial efficiencies of protein and fat by regression methods. Proc. 9th Symp. on Energy Metabolism, Lillehammer, EAAP Publ. No. **29**, 138 (1982)
[29] THORBEK, G., A. CHWALIBOG and S. HENCKEL: Beretning 563. National Institute of Animal Science. Copenhagen. 114pp. (1984)
[30] VERMOREL, M. and J. KELLER: Energetic utilization by growing rats of the principal cereals as components of diets balanced with respect to protein and aminoacids. Proc. 4th Symp. on Energy Metabolism, Warsaw, EAAP Publ. No. **12**, 387 (1969)
[31] WALKER, D. M. and B. W. NORTON: J. Agric. Sci., Camb. **77**, 363 (1971)

Received 28 April 1987

Address of authors:

Dr. J. F. AGUILERA and Dr. C. PRIETO
Estación Experimental del Zaidín (C. S. I. C)
Granada
Profesor Albareda 1
Apartado 419
Spain

Arch. Anim. Nutr., Berlin 37 (1897) 10, 895–903

Institut für tropische Landwirtschaftt der Karl-Marx-Universität Leipzig,
Fachgruppe Tierproduktion
(Leiter: Dr. sc. S. LEGEL)

S. LEGEL und A. A. RUKANTABULA

Untersuchungen zur Beeinflussung des Rohnährstoffgehaltes von Futtermitteln tropischer Regionen während der Lagerung unter extremen Klimabedingungen

2. Mitteilung

Wirkung unter ariden wechselnden Klimabedingungen

1. Einleitung

In tropischen und subtropischen Regionen sind Futtermittel wesentlich intensiveren klimatischen Einflußfaktoren ausgesetzt als in gemäßigten Zonen. Aus den genannten Gründen ist mit hohen Substanz- und Nährstoffverlusten von gelagerten Futtermitteln zu rechnen. Da bisher dazu wenig Ergebnisse vorliegen, wurde unter simulierten Klimabedingungen die Wirkung von extremen Temperaturen und extrem hoher oder geringer relativer Luftfeuchtigkeit auf Veränderungen des Nährstoffgehaltes charakteristischer Futtermittel untersucht. Begründung und Zielstellung der vorgenommenen Versuche wurden in Verbindung mit einer Literaturrecherche in der 1. Mitt. (LEGEL u. a., 1987) genannt, in welcher auch die Beeinflussung des Rohnährstoffgehaltes von Futtermitteln unter humiden konstanten Klimabedingungen dargestellt wurde, während sich die vorliegende Mitteilung mit der Wirkung unter ariden wechselnden Klimabedingungen beschäftigt.

2. Material und Methode

Die Untersuchungen zur Wirkung von ariden wechselnden Klimabedingungen wurden über einen Zeitraum von 150 Tagen (22. 10. 81 bis 22. 3. 82) im Institut für tropische Landwirtschaft der Karl-Marx-Universität Leipzig durchgeführt. Die erforderlichen Klimabedingungen wurden mit Hilfe eines Klimaschrankes simuliert. Das aride Klima mit typischem Wechsel von hohen Tages- und tiefen Nachttemperaturen und den damit verbundenen Veränderungen der relativen Luftfeuchtigkeit (RL) wurde durch einen 12stündigen Wechsel von jeweils 40 °C und 15 % RL sowie 10 °C und 95 % RL simuliert. Die Behandlung der untersuchten Futtermittel sowie deren chemische Analyse wurden in der 1. Mitt. (LEGEL u. a., 1987) beschrieben.

3. Ergebnisse und Diskussion

Die Ergebnisse der Veränderungen im Trockensubstanzgehalt, Rohnährstoffgehalt, Reinproteingehalt und der Fettqualitätsparameter werden in Tab. 1 (Maiskörner), Tab. 2 (Sojaextraktionsschrot) und Tab. 3 (Luzerne-Trockengrün) dargestellt.

Tabelle 1 (Table 1)

Veränderung der Rohnährstoffgehalte und Fettqualitätsparameter von Maiskörnern während einer 5monatigen Lagerung bei Wechselklima sowie Signifikanz der ermittelten Differenzen bei $\alpha < 0{,}05$*

(Variability of the crude nutrient content and the parameters of fat quality of maize during a period of 5 months storing under changed climatic conditions and the statistical calculation of differences by $p < 0.05$)*

Ermittelte Parameter (Parameters)		Lagerdauer in Tagen und Datum der Probeentnahme [Duration of storing (days) and date of taking samples] 0 22. 10. 81	30 23. 11. 81	60 23. 12. 81	90 21. 1. 82	120 22. 2. 82	150 22. 3. 82
Originalsubstanz (Original matter)	(g)	100,00	94,4	102,6	92,3	106,0	90,5
Trockensubstanz (Dry matter)	(%)	85,8[a]	89,6[b]	83,8[c]	91,0[d]	88,5[e]	92,6[f]
Gehalt in der Trockensubstanz: (Content in the dry matter):							
Rohprotein (Crude protein)	(%)	9,4[a]	9,6[b]	9,2[a]	9,8[b]	9,8[b]	10,2[c]
Reinprotein (True protein)	(%)	8,9[a]	8,7[b]	8,6[b]	9,3[c]	9,0[a]	8,4[d]
Rohfett (Crude fat)	(%)	4,7[ab]	4,3[c]	4,5[bc]	4,9[a]	3,4[d]	4,5[bc]
NFE (NFE)	(%)	81,7	81,7	81,9	80,7	82,0	80,6
Rohfaser (Crude fibre)	(%)	2,9	2,6	2,9	2,9	2,8	2,7
Rohasche (Ash)	(%)	1,4[a]	1,7[b]	1,5[a]	1,7[b]	2,0[c]	2,0[c]
Jodzahl (Iodine No.)		118,5			101,2		97,8
Säurezahl (Acid No.)		137,5			82,2		78,3
Verseifungszahl (Saponification No.)		190,3			179,2		184,3

* Zahlen mit gleichen Buchstaben innerhalb einer Zeile sind nicht miteinander signifikant
Zahlen mit verschiedenen Buchstaben innerhalb einer Zeile sind miteinander signifikant
(Differences of numbers with equal letters within the line are not significant
Differences of numbers with different letters within the line are significant)

Trockensubstanz

Die drei Futtermittel zeigten keine deutliche Tendenz in der Veränderung des Trockensubstanzgehaltes unter wechselnden Klimabedingungen. Nach 150 Lagerungstagen lag der TS-Gehalt bei allen Futtermitteln allerdings weit über dem Ausgangswert und stimmte in der Tendenz mit Ergebnissen von CZERKAWSKI (1967) überein.

Roh- und Reinprotein

Beim Mais war keine wesentliche Veränderung im Roh- und Reinproteingehalt und in der absoluten Proteinmenge festzustellen. Der Proteingehalt zeigte jedoch eine sehr geringe, aber tendenzielle Zunahme. Sojaextraktionsschrot und Luzerne-Trockengrün

Tabelle 2 (Table 2)

Veränderung der Rohnährstoffgehalte und Fettqualitätsparameter von Sojaextraktraktionsschrot während einer 5monatigen Lagerung bei Wechselklima sowie Signifikanz der ermittelten Differenzen bei $\alpha < 0,05$*

(Variability of the crude nutrient content and the parameters of fat quality of soya oil meal during a period of 5 months storing under changed climatic conditions and the statistical calculation of differences by $p < 0.05$)*

Ermittelte Parameter (Parameters)		Lagerdauer in Tagen und Datum der Probeentnahme [Duration of storing (days) and date of taking samples]					
		0 22. 10. 81	30 23. 11. 81	60 23. 12. 81	90 21. 1. 82	120 22. 2. 82	150 22. 3. 82
Originalsubstanz (Original matter)	(g)	100,0	92,5	106,2	86,4	100,4	84,4
Trockensubstanz (Dry matter)	(%)	$86,3^{a}$	$91,8^{b}$	$79,0^{c}$	$91,4^{d}$	$87,9^{e}$	$93,1^{f}$
Gehalt in der Trockensubstanz: (Content in the dry matter):							
Rohprotein (Crude protein)	(%)	$48,2^{a}$	$45,6^{b}$	$47,7^{ac}$	$47,5^{c}$	$51,8^{d}$	$48,4^{a}$
Reinprotein (True protein)	(%)	$44,4^{a}$	$42,4^{b}$	$46,4^{c}$	$45,6^{d}$	$49,4^{e}$	$45,6^{d}$
Rohfett (Crude fat)	(%)	$1,1^{a}$	$0,9^{bc}$	$1,0^{abc}$	$0,9^{c}$	$0,9^{c}$	$0,9^{c}$
NFE (NFE)	(%)	35,2	35,2	33,8	32,2	29,8	32,8
Rohfaser (Crude fibre)	(%)	$9,0^{b}$	$11,6^{b}$	$10,7^{c}$	$12,2^{d}$	$10,1^{a}$	$10,6^{c}$
Rohasche (Ash)	(%)	$6,6^{a}$	$6,9^{ab}$	$6,8^{ab}$	$7,2^{b}$	$7,4^{b}$	$7,3^{b}$
Jodzahl (Iodine No.)		116,5			101,1		
Säurezahl (Acid No.)		81,0			50,2		
Verseifungszahl (Saponification No.)		59,4			187,3		

* = siehe Tab. 1 (see Table 1)

wiesen große Schwankungen im Roh- und Reinproteingehalt und in der gesamten Proteinmenge auf. Der Wert der gesamten Proteinmenge lag jedoch bei den beiden Futtermitteln unter dem Anfangswert.

Rohfett

Der Rohfettgehalt und die Gesamtfettmenge blieben beim Mais bis zum Ende der Lagerung im allgemeinen unverändert. Beim Sojaextraktionsschrot trat nach 90 und bei Luzerne-Trockengrün nach 60 Lagertagen eine deutliche Abnahme des Rohfettgehaltes auf. In der Folgezeit blieb er bis Versuchsende konstant. Aus diesen Ergebnissen ist festzustellen, daß die Lagerstabilität des Fettes unter 12stündiger Wechseltemperatur und ebenso wechselnder relativer Luftfeuchtigkeit beim Luzerne-Trockengrün am geringsten und beim Mais am höchsten war.

Tabelle 3 (Table 3)

Veränderung der Rohnährstoffgehalte von Luzerne-Trockengrün während einer 5monatigen Lagerung bei Wechselklima sowie Signifikanz der ermittelten Differenzen bei $\alpha < 0{,}05$*

(Variability of the crude nutrient content of alfalfa meal during a period of 5 months under changed climatic conditions and the statistical calculation of differences by $p < 0.05$)*

Ermittelte Parameter (Parameters)		Lagerdauer in Tagen und Datum der Probeentenahme [Duration of storing (days) and date of taking samples] 0 22. 10. 81	30 23. 11. 81	60 23. 12. 81	90 21. 1. 82	120 22. 2. 82	150 22. 3. 82
Originalsubstanz (Original matter)	(g)	100,0	92,4	102,8	84,8	96,9	81,0
Trockensubstanz (Dry matter)	(%)	88,1^{a}	91,6^{b}	78,8^{c}	91,5^{b}	88,1^{a}	93,5^{d}
Gehalt in der Trockensubstanz: (Content in the dry matter):							
Rohprotein (Crude protein)	(%)	19,8^{a}	17,4^{b}	20,6^{c}	19,0^{d}	21,1^{e}	17,6^{b}
Reinprotein (True protein)	(%)	14,7^{a}	12,4^{b}	17,5^{c}	16,6^{d}	17,0^{e}	15,0^{f}
Rohfett (Crude fat)	(%)	2,6^{a}	2,0^{b}	1,6^{c}	1,7^{c}	1,8^{c}	1,8^{c}
NFE (NFE)	(%)	38,7	38,0	33,4	32,6	32,1	36,5
(Rohfaser) Crude fibre)	(%)	27,0^{b}	31,2^{b}	31,8^{bd}	32,6^{c}	32,1^{cd}	32,6^{cd}
Rohasche (Ash)	(%)	11,9^{a}	11,4^{b}	12,6^{c}	14,1^{d}	13,0^{e}	11,6^{f}

* = siehe Tab. 1 (see Table 1)

N-freie Extraktstoffe

Die Veränderung des NFE-Gehaltes war beim Mais nur geringfügig. Nach 150tägiger Lagerung lag der NFE-Gehaltswert knapp unter dem Ausgangswert. Beim Sojaextraktionsschrot und Luzerne-Trockengrün wurde ab 60. Lagerungstag eine nennenswerte Verminderung des NFE-Gehaltes festgestellt. Die eingetretenen Verluste an N-freien Extraktstoffen bei Sojaextraktionsschrot und Luzerne-Trockengrün können nach FRANCIS und WOOD (1980) möglicherweise auf den pilzlichen Abbau der Kohlenhydrate zurückgeführt werden.

Rohfaser

Der Rohfasergehalt blieb bei Mais bis zum Versuchsende unverändert. Bei Sojaextraktionsschrot und Luzerne-Trockengrün unterlag er Schwankungen, zeigte aber in der Tendenz eine Zunahme. Diese Zunahme kann eine Folge der gleichzeitigen trockensubstanzbezogenen Abnahme des Rohfettgehaltes gewesen sein.

Tabelle 4 (Table 4)

Veränderung der Gehalte und der Menge an „Energetischen Futtereinheiten, Rind" (EFr) während einer 150tägigen Lagerung von Futtermitteln bei humidem Konstant- und aridem Wechselklima

[Variability of the contents and the quantity of the "energetic feed units/ruminant" (EFUr) of feedstuffs during a period of 150 days storing under humid constant and arid changed climatic conditions]

Ermittelte Parameter (Parameters)	Futtermittel (Feedstuff) Maiskörner (Maize) K*	W**	Sojaextraktions-schrot (Soya oil meal) K	W	Luzerne-Trockengrün (Alfalfa meal) K	W
EFr/ 1 kg TS***: (EFUr/ kg dry matter):						
vor Lagerung (before storing)	788	791	642	636	432	429
nach Lagerung (after storing)	707	781	612	626	398	418
EFr in TS-Menge: (EFUr in the amount of the dry matter):						
im Ausgangsmaterial (in the initial material)	68,9	67,9	57,4	54,9	39,9	37,8
im Endmaterial (in the final material)	57,6	65,5	46,4	49,2	32,1	31,7
EFr-Verluste während der Lagerzeit in % (EFUr-losses during the storage time in %)	16,4	3,5	19,2	10,4	19,5	16,1

* K = Konstantklima, humid (Constant climate, humid)
** W = Wechselklima, arid (Changed climate, arid)
*** = Trockensubstanz

Rohasche

Der Rohaschegehalt und die gesamte Rohaschemenge zeigten mit fortschreitender Lagerungsdauer einen tendenziellen Anstieg. Dieser Anstieg war beim Mais ausgeprägter als bei den anderen Futtermitteln.

Fettqualitätsparameter

Die Jodzahl zeigte beim Mais und Sojaextraktionsschrot eine lineare Abnahme. Diese Ergebnisse deuten daraufhin, daß die Fettoxydation stattgefunden hat, womit ein Fettverderbsprozeß eingeleitet wurde. Hinsichtlich der Veränderung der Säurezahl und der Verseifungszahl können keine zielgerichteten Aussagen gemacht werden.

Organoleptische Prüfung

Nach 60 Lagerungstagen trat ein muffiger Geruch bei allen drei Futtermitteln auf. Beim Mais blieb der Geruch bis zum Versuchsende nur leicht muffig, während bei den übrigen Futtermitteln ein stark muffiger Geruch am Ende der Versuchsdauer festzustellen war. Nach 60 Lagertagen wurde ebenfalls bei allen drei Futtermitteln eine Abweichung in der Farbe festgestellt. An Versuchsende waren die Futtermittel mit grau-grünem Schimmelbelag überzogen.

4. Gegenüberstellung der Ergebnisse unter konstanten und wechselnden Klimabedingungen

Während eine deutliche Abnahme des TS-Gehaltes bei allen drei Futtermitteln unter Konstantklima zu verzeichnen war, zeichnet sich der TS-Gehalt der untersuchten Futtermittel bei Wechselklima durch unregelmäßigen Verlauf aus. Nach 150tägiger Lagerung lag aber der TS-Gehalt weit über dem Ausgangswert. Am Versuchsend wurde jedoch in beiden Versuchsserien ein Rückgang in der gesamten Trockensubstanzmenge festgestellt. Es war eine relative Zunahme im Roh- und Reinproteingehalt beim Mais unter Konstantklima zu registrieren. Beim Wechselklima blieb der Roh- und Reinproteingehalt im allgemeinen unverändert. Sojaextraktionsschrot und Luzerne-Trockengrün wiesen in beiden Versuchsserien Unregelmäßigkeiten auf.

Der Fett- und NFE-Gehalt wurden am meisten unter Konstantbedingungen betroffen. Der Rohfettgehalt nahm bei allen drei Futtermitteln sehr stark ab. Unter Wechselbedingungen veränderte sich der Rohfettgehalt beim Mais nicht. Er verringerte sich aber beim Sojaextraktionsschrot und Luzerne-Trockengrün geringfügig. Der NFE-Gehalt verringerte sich bei Sojaextraktionsschrot und Luzerne-Trockengrün unter beiden Klimabedingungen. Diese Verringerung war bei Konstantklima höher als bei Wechselklima.

Rohfaser- und Rohaschegehalt veränderten sich beim Mais sowohl unter Konstantklima als auch unter Wechselklima nur unwesentlich. Rohfaser und Rohasche zeichneten sich bei Sojaextraktionsschrot und Luzerne-Trockengrün durch eine steigende Tendenz bei beiden Versuchsarten aus.

Die Jodzahl ging beim Mais und Sojaextraktionsschrot bei beiden Versuchsarten tendenziell zurück. Der Rückgang war nach gleicher Lagerdauer bei Konstantklima stärker als bei Wechselklima. Es war ein geringer Rückgang der Säurezahl beim Mais unter Konstantklima zu beobachten. Der gleiche Kennwert erhöhte sich bei Sojaextraktionsschrot nur wenig. Unter Wechselklimabedingungen verringerte sich der Kennwert sowohl beim Mais als auch beim Sojaextraktionsschrot.

Die Unterschiede zwischen Konstant- und Wechselklima können in der unterschiedlichen Lagertemperatur und relativen Luftfeuchtigkeit begründet sein. Das Auftreten von Phasen mit tiefen Temperaturen und geringer relativer Luftfeuchtigkeit bei Wechselklima hat vermutlich den negativen Einfluß andauernder hoher Temperaturen und hoher relativer Luftfeuchtigkeit gemildert.

Die nach einer jeweiligen Lagerungszeit von 150 Tagen aufgetretenen Verluste an EFr während der simulierten Klimabedingungen sind in Tab. 4 aufgeführt. Die geringsten Verluste wurden bei Maiskörnern ermittelt, und zwar unter beiden Klimabedingungen. Bei allen drei untersuchten Futtermitteln konnten unter humiden konstanten Klimabedingungen erheblich höhere Verluste registriert werden als unter ariden wechselnden Klimabedingungen.

Besonders deutlich war die Differenz der Verluste zwischen beiden Klimabedingungen bei Maiskörnern.

Aus dem vorliegenden Versuch geht hervor, daß die Lagerung von Mais, Sojaextraktionsschrot und Luzerne-Trockengrün unter konstanter hoher Temperatur und hoher relativer Luftfeuchtigkeit mit einer wesentlichen Verringerung des TS-Gehaltes, des Rohfettgehaltes und des NFE-Gehaltes sowie einer Beeinträchtigung der Geruchs- und Farbeigenschaften verbunden ist. Sollen keine anderen Maßnahmen ergriffen werden, so dürfen die zu Untersuchungen herangezogenen Futtermittel unter Verhältnissen, die den Versuchsbedingungen ähnlich sind, nicht über 30 Tage gelagert werden. Bei einer Verfütterung von über 30 Tage gelagerten Futtermitteln müssen die eingetretenen Veränderungen berücksichtigt werden.

Bei der Lagerung der untersuchten Futtermittel unter einem 12stündigen Wechsel von Temperatur und relativer Luftfeuchtigkeit bleibt Mais in seinem Rohnährstoffgehalt fast unverändert.

Sojaextraktionsschrot und Luzerne-Trockengrün weisen aber signifikante Verluste im Fett- und NFE-Gehalt auf. Nach 60 Lagerungstagen treten bei allen drei Futtermitteln mikrobielle Veränderungen auf, so daß dies, trotz geringen Verlustes der Rohnährstoffe, als lagerbegrenzender Faktor anzusehen ist.

Generell sind in ariden Gebieten mit typischem Wechsel der Temperatur und relativen Luftfeuchtigkeit bessere Lagerungsbedingungen gegeben als unter konstanten humiden Bedingungen.

Die in dieser Arbeit erzielten Versuchsergebnisse sollen durch solche aus Lagerungsversuchen unter praktischen tropischen Bedingungen und durch Verwendung von Futtermitteln, die in der chemischen Zusammensetzung und physikalischen Struktur von denen der untersuchten Futtermittel abweichen, ergänzt werden. Künftig sind mikroskopische Untersuchungen hinsichtlich der Bakterien- und Pilzbestimmung und deren Besatz einzubeziehen, um die Beziehungen zwischen der organoleptischen Prüfung, dem Rohnährstoffgehalt und der mikrobiellen Veränderung besser zu verdeutlichen.

Zusammenfassung

In Fortführung von Untersuchungen zur Beeinflussung des Rohnährstoffgehaltes durch humide konstante Klimabedingungen sind in der vorliegenden Arbeit die Veränderungen im Rohnährstoffgehalt von Mais, Sojaextraktionsschrot und Luzerne-Trockengrün unter ariden wechselnden Klimabedingungen ermittelt worden. Über einen Zeitraum von 150 Tagen wurde in einer Klimakammer ein arides Wüstenklima mit einem 12stündigen Wechsel von jeweils 40 °C und 15 % relativer Luftfeuchtigkeit (RL) sowie 10 °C und 95 % RL simuliert.

Alle drei Futtermittel zeigten keine deutliche Tendenz in der Veränderung des Trockensubstanzgehaltes. Er lag am Ende der Lagerung jedoch über den Ausgangswerten. Der Gehalt an Roh- und Reinprotein zeigte bei allen Futtermitteln eine geringfügige tendenzielle Zunahme und unterlag bei Sojaextraktionsschrot und Luzerne-Trockengrün großen Schwankungen. Bei Sojaextraktionsschrot trat nach 90 Tagen und bei Luzerne-Trockengrün nach 60 Tagen ein deutlicher Abfall des Rohfettgehaltes auf.

Der NFE-Gehalt verminderte sich bei allen Futtermitteln, der Rohfasergehalt unterlag Schwankungen.

Ohne wesentliche Veränderungen der Rohnährstoffgehalte und organoleptischen Parameter können die untersuchten Futtermittel unter ariden wechselnden Klimabedingungen 60 Tage und unter humiden konstanten Klimabedingungen 30 Tage gelagert werden.

Резюме

С. Легель и А. А. Рукантабула

Исследования по влиянию на содержание сырых питательных веществ кормов тропических районов во время хранения под экстремальными климатическими условиями. 2-ое сообщ.: Действие при аридных переменных условиях климата

В продолжении работ по влиянию содержания сырых питательных веществ при гумидных постоянных условиях климата сообщается в данной стате об изменениях содержания сырых питательных веществ кукурузы, соевого шрота и зелёной муки из люцерны при аридных переменных условиях климата. За 150 дней симулировался в климатической камере аридный климат пустынь с 12-часовой переменой от 40 °С и 15 % относительной влажности воздуха с 10 °С и 95 % относительной влажности воздуха.

Содержание сухого в-ва этих трёх кормов практически не изменилось, но в конце хранения находилось свыше исходных данных. Содержания сырого и чистого протеинов в тенденции незначительно повышались у всех кормов, но у соевого шрота и у зелёной муки из люцерны наблюдали широкие колебания. Значительное снижение содержания сырого жира определено после 90 дней у соевого шрота и после 60 дней у зелёной муки из люцерны. Содержание БЭВа сокращалось у всех кормов, а относительно содержания клечатки определилось широкое колебание.

Исследуемые корма можно хранить 60 дней при аридных переменных условиях климата и 30 дней при гумидных постоянных климатических условиях, без того, чтобы содéржание сырых питательных веществ и органолептических параметров значительно изменились.

Summary

S. Legel and A. A. Rukantabula

Studies of the influence of the crude nutrient content of feedstuffs in tropical regions during the storage under extreme climatic conditions. 2. Effects under changing arid climatic conditions

In continuation of studies of the influentiation of the crude nutrient content by constantly humid climatic conditions, this paper describes changes in the crude nutrient content of maize, soybean oilmeal and alfalfa meal ascertained under changing arid conditions. Over a period of 150 days an arid desert climate was simulated in a climatic chamber with a 12-hourly change from 40 °C and 15 % air humidity to 10 °C and 95 % air humidity.

None of the three feedstuffs showed a clear tendency in the change of the dry matter content. At the end of the storage period it was, however, higher than the original values. For all feedstuffs the crude and pure protein content showed an insignificantly increasing tendency and underwent big variations with soybean oilmeal and alfalfa meal. There was a distinct decrease of the crude fat content of soybean oilmeal after 90 days and of alfalfa meal after 60 days.

The NFE content decreased in all feedstuffs, the crude fibre content underwent variations.

The feedstuffs studied may be stored without essential changes of the crude nutrient content and the organoleptic parameters for 60 days under changing arid climatic conditions and for 30 days under constant humid climatic conditions.

Literaturverzeichnis

[1] Czerkawski, J. W.: Brit. Journ. Nutrit., **21**, 599 (1967)
[2] Francis, B. J. und J. F. Wood: Tropical Science, **22**, 219 (1980)
[3] Legel, S., A. A. Rukantabula und Ch. Geissler: Arch. Tierernähr. **37**, 371 (1987)

Eingegangen: 5. September 1986

Anschrift der Autoren:

Dr. sc. S. Legel und Dipl. Agr.-Ing. A. A. Rukantabula
Institut für tropische Landwirtschaft der
Karl-Marx-Universität Leipzig
Fachgruppe Tierproduktion
Raschwitzer Str. 16
Markkleeberg
DDR - 7113

Arch. Anim. Nutr., Berlin 37 (1987) 10, 905–953

Jahrestagung der Gesellschaft für Ernährung in der DDR, Sektion Tierernährung, vom 1.–3. Oktober 1986 in Neubrandenburg

(Kurzreferate)

Einführung

Im Namen des Vorstandes begrüßte der Vorsitzende der Sektion Tierernährung, Prof. Dr. S. Poppe, die 158 Teilnehmer der Tagung, die zu dem Generalthema „Nichttraditionelle Futtermittel – Futterwert und Einsatzmöglichkeiten" durchgeführt wurde.

In Würdigung der großen Verdienste, die sich Oskar Kellner durch seine umfangreichen wissenschaftlichen und praktischen Forschungsarbeiten im Hinblick auf die Profilierung Tierernährung und -fütterung als eigenständige Wissenschaftsdisziplin erworben hat, wurde anläßlich seines 75. Todestages von Prof. Dr. R. Schiemann ein Gedenkvortrag gehalten, der nachstehend ungekürzt abgedruckt ist. Vor Beginn des Tagungsprogrammes erfolgte die Auszeichnung von Dr. sc. O. Simon (Berlin) für seine Forschungsarbeiten auf dem Gebiet des Eiweißumsatzes bei Monogastriden mit dem Arthur-Scheunert-Preis der Gesellschaft für Ernährung durch den Vorsitzenden der Gesellschaft, Prof. Dr. G. Gebhardt. Die Vortragstagung war auf die Schwerpunkte

- Strohaufbereitung und -Einsatz
- Exkrementaufbereitung und -Einsatz
- Eiweißmischsilageproduktion und -Einsatz

und aus aktuellem Anlaß auf den Schwerpunkt

- Möglichkeiten der Grünfutterkonservierung ausgerichtet.

Darüber hinaus fand zum Tagungsprogramm und zu freien Themen eine rege Posterdiskussion statt (insgesamt 45 Poster), die durch ein Podiumsgespräch, das durch kompetente Fachwissenschaftler geleitet wurde, eine zusammenfassende Wertung erfuhr.

Forschungszentrum für Tierproduktion Dummerstorf-Rostock der Akademie der Landwirtschaftswissenschaften der DDR, Bereich Tierernährung „Oskar Kellner“

R. SCHIEMANN

Zum 75. Todestag von OSKAR KELLNER

Am 22. September 1986 jährte sich zum 75. Mal der Tag, an dem Oskar KELLNER durch Herzversagen in Karlsruhe auf der 31. Hauptversammlung des Verbandes der Landwirtschaftlichen Versuchsstationen Deutschlands im Alter von 60 Jahren verstarb. „Er war“, wie F. HONCAMP (Die landwirtschaftliche Versuchsstationen 76 (1912), S. III–XLIV) in seinem Nachruf für Oskar KELLNER berichtet, „schaffensfreudig und in einer gehobenen Stimmung noch am Tage vor seinem Tode nach Karlsruhe gefahren. Ahnte er doch, daß man seitens des Verbandes landwirtschaftlicher Versuchsstationen eine Ehrung für ihn plante, die bisher noch keinem Verbandsmitglied zuteil geworden war, nämlich die Ernennung zum Ehrenvorsitzenden des Verbandes. Voll von froher Hoffnung und kühnen Plänen hat er noch während der langen Eisenbahnfahrt zu verschiedenen mitfahrenden Kollegen über seine Versuchspläne für die nächsten Jahre gesprochen.“

Wir wollen uns zunächst einige Daten seines Lebensweges vergegenwärtigen.

Oskar KELLNER wurde am 13. Mai 1851 in der schlesischen Kleinstadt Tillowitz geboren. Über sein Elternhaus ist uns nichts bekannt. Im Jahre 1871 bestand er das Abiturientenexamen am Realgymnasium in Neiße, nachdem er den Schulbesuch wegen Teilnahme am deutsch-französischen Krieg 1870/71 für etwa 1 Jahr hatte unterbrechen müssen. Anschließend studierte er in Breslau und Leipzig Naturwissenschaften unter besonderer Berücksichtigung der Chemie und absolvierte bereits nach 3jährigem Studium (1874) das Doktorexamen an der Philosophischen Fakultät der Universität Leipzig. Seine Promotionsarbeit „Über einige chemische Vorgänge bei der Keimung von pisum sativum“, deren Ergebnisse in der Zeitschrift „Die landwirtschaftlichen Versuchsstationen“ (Bd. 7, 1874, S. 408) schon im gleichen Jahr publiliziert wurden, fällt bereits in das Gebiet der Agrikulturchemie. Nach dem Studium nahm er eine Tätigkeit als Assistent am Tierchemischen Institut der Landwirtschaftlichen Akademie in Proskau (Schlesien) bei dem Agrikulturchemiker Hugo WEISKE auf, der sich besonders mit tierphysiologischen Untersuchungen und fütterungstechnischen Fragen befaßte. Die 2jährige Assistentenzeit bei WEISKE hat den wissenschaftlichen Werdegang KELLNERS sicher wesentlich beeinflußt. Aus dieser relativ kurzen Zeit bezeugen 10 Publikationen, mit welcher Intensität und Akribie KELLNER gearbeitet hat, wobei er der experimentellen Arbeit stets eine wesentliche Bedeutung beimaß. Zum besseren Verständnis des Entwicklungsweges möchte ich einige Arbeiten KELLNERS aus dieser Zeit anführen:

- Die Veränderungen ganzer Körper im Verdauungsapparat des Kalbes
- Versuche über den Einfluß des Scherens bei Schafen auf die Ausnutzung des Futters sowie auf den Stickstoffumsatz
- Zusammensetzung verschiedener Futtermittel
- Versuche über Verwertung animalischer Futtermittel durch Pflanzenfresser
- Versuche über die Aufenthaltsdauer des Futters im Verdauungsapparat der Tiere, insbesondere des Schafes

Neben der vielfältigen Versuchstätigkeit hatte KELLNER in Proskau auch umfangreiche Vorlesungsverpflichtungen und trat bereits als junger Assistent auf der 48. Versammlung deutscher Naturforscher und Ärzte (1875 in Graz) mit 2 Vorträgen vor die Öffentlichkeit. 1876 ging KELLNER an die Landwirtschaftliche Versuchsstation Hohenheim, um hier bei Emil VON WOLFF, einem der Begründer der deutschen Tierernährungswissenschaft und ersten Direktor der Landwirtschaftlichen Versuchsstation in Möckern (1852–54), Assistent zu werden. Bedeutsam war hier für KELLNER die Verbindung der Landwirtschaftlichen Versuchsstation mit der Hohenheimer Akademie, um sich gründliche Einblicke in die verschiedensten Zweige der Landwirtschaftswissenschaften zu verschaffen.

In der 5jährigen Tätigkeit in Hohenheim hat sich KELLNER wiederum in erster Linie mit fütterungstechnischen und ernährungsphysiologischen Fragen beschäftigt. Er hat aber auch gemäß der agrikulturchemischen Arbeitsbreite pflanzenphysiologische Probleme, insbesondere Probleme des N-Umsatzes, bearbeitet. Die aus dieser Zeit in Hohenheim resultierende große Zahl wissenschaftlich gut fundierter Publikationen – es sind mehr als 30 – und Vorträge auf fachlichen Tagungen führten dazu, daß KELLNER sehr früh internationale Anerkennung fand. So erhielt er 1881 als 29jähriger eine ehrenvolle Berufung als Professor für Agrikulturchemie an die Kaiserlich-japanische Universität in Tokio.

Bevor ich auf die Tätigkeit in Japan zu sprechen komme, möchte ich noch kurz auf eine Arbeit aus der Hohenheimer Zeit eingehen, die mir als besonders bedeutsam erscheint, nämlich die Arbeit „Zusammenhang zwischen Muskeltätigkeit und Stoffzerfall im tierischen Organismus", die in 2 Mitteilungen („Landwirtschaftliche Jahrbücher", Bd. 8 (1879) und Bd. 9 (1880)) erschienen ist. In umfangreichen Bilanzversuchen mit Pferden, deren Arbeitsleistung mit Hilfe eines Bremsgöpelwerkes (Pferdedynamometer) gemessen wurde, konnte KELLNER nachweisen, daß – entgegen der vorherrschenden Meinung, daß Eiweiß für die Erzeugung von Muskelkraft zersetzt werden müsse – bei reichlicher Zufuhr von Kohlenhydraten keine Erhöhung der N-Bilanz auch bei starker Arbeitsleistung auftrat und damit die Vertretbarkeit der Nährstoffe Protein und Kohlenhydrate nach ihrem physiologischen Energielieferungsvermögen bewiesen war. Hervorzuheben ist die von KELLNER aus diesen Arbeiten vorausschauend gezogene Schlußfolgerung zur Bedeutung der Messung des Energieumsatzes im tierischen Organismus. So schreibt er 1880: „Unsere Versuche legen fernerhin dar, wie richtig es wäre, die Verbrennungswärme einzelner Komponenten der Nahrung sowie namentlich ganzer Nahrungsmittel festzustellen, da die genauen Mischungsverhältnisse bestimmter chemischer Verbindungen in den einzelnen zur Ernährung dienenden Materialien unserer Erkenntnis noch sehr fern liegen.

Spezifische Funktionen in der Ernährung kommen allem Anschein nach nur den Eiweißkörpern, deren Derivaten und einzelnen Mineralstoffen zu. Diese gesamte Menge der stickstofffreien Nahrungsbestandteile dagegen scheint nur einem Zweck zu dienen, den J. v. LIEBIG im Auge hatte, als er sie als Respirationsmittel bezeichnete. Für die Bestimmung des Nährwertes dieser Stoffgruppen hat die Ermittlung der Verbrennungswärme einen unbestreitbaren Wert, sie bildet vielleicht den richtigen Maßstab der Wertschätzung."

Diese Feststellung liegt 3 Jahre vor der Zeit, in der RUBNER seine grundlegenden Untersuchungen über den Energieumsatz, so auch das Gesetz von der isodynamen Vertretbarkeit der Nährstoffe im tierischen Organismus (1883), veröffentlichte. Aus der Publikation zum Muskelstoffwechsel ist für KELLNERS spätere Arbeiten noch eine Bemerkung wesentlich. Er stellte fest, daß man gegenwärtig noch weit davon entfernt sei, Wertigkeitsverhältnisse der Nahrungsbestandteile für bestimmte Produktionsrichtungen aufstellen zu können.

Nach Hohenheim folgte eine 12jährige Tätigkeit in Japan, die nach anfänglichen Schwierigkeiten des Einlebens und Durchsetzens didaktischer Prinzipien bei der Ausbildung nach eigenen Aussagen gegenüber Kollegen zu der schönsten Zeit seines Lebens gehörte. In Japan fand er auch seine Lebensgefährtin und gründete eine Familie. Über das Schicksal der beiden Kinder, einer Tochter und eines Sohnes, ist uns Näheres leider nicht bekannt, außer der Erinnerung an einen kurzen Besuch der Tochter im Oskar-Kellner-Institut 1958, bei dem sie die Urkunde über die Verleihung der Ehrendoktorwürde der medizinischen Fakultät in Breslau an ihren Vater, die am 3. 8. 1911, also wenige Wochen vor seinem Tode, stattfand, uns übergab. Aus der ersten Zeit in Japan möchte ich zur weiteren Charakterisierung der Persönlichkeit Oskar KELLNERS eine Episode einflechten, die von F. HONCAMP wie folgt beschrieben wird:

„Er selbst hat uns einmal erzählt, daß unter seinem Amtsvorgänger, einem Amerikaner oder Engländer, der Brauch eingerissen sei, daß die Studenten zum Examen zugelassen wurden, ohne sich durch längere praktische Arbeiten im Laboratorium die genügenden manuellen Fertigkeiten angeeignet zu haben. Hiermit räumte KELLNER sofort und gründlich auf. Er wußte sehr wohl, daß theoretische Kenntnisse zwar unbedingt und unerlässliche Vorbedingungen waren, daß aber diese allein noch nicht den jungen Agrikulturchemiker machten und daß mit dem eigentlichen theoretischen Wissen auch eine gründliche praktische Ausbildung unbedingt Hand in Hand gehen mußte. Trotz der Beschwerde seiner Studenten bei KELLNERS vorgesetzter Behörde, beharrte er bei seiner Forderung, und er setzte sie auch glücklich durch. Dieses unbeugsame, starre Festhalten an dem einmal für richtig Erkannten, wie dies KELLNER eigen war, hat aber vielleicht auch nicht zum wenigsten mit dazu beigetragen, daß er sich von Anfang an in Japan eine sichere Position zu schaffen wußte. Ganz zweifelsohne hat er sogleich den japanischen Charakter richtig erkannt und seine Studenten in einer Art und Weise zu nehmen gewußt, die ihm für alle Zeiten die Liebe und Verehrung seiner japanischen Schüler gesichert hat."

Neben der Lehrtätigkeit hat KELLNER in Japan umfangreiche, für die japanische Landwirtschaft außerordentlich bedeutsame Forschungsarbeiten in Angriff genommen und gleichzeitig das landwirtschaftliche Versuchswesen grundlegend reorganisiert. Folgende Problemkomplexe wurden von ihm in Japan vorrangig bearbeitet:

- Düngung und Kultur des Reisanbaues (Reis als wichtigste Ernährungsgrundlage der Japaner)
- Chemische Untersuchung von Ackerböden
- Zusammensetzung und Qualität für Japan typischer Futtermittel

- Ernährung der Seidenraupen (Seidenproduktion als für Japan ökonomisch sehr wichtiger Produktionszweig)

Aus den Ergebnissen zum letztgenannten Forschungskomplex ist der experimentelle Befund sehr bedeutsam, daß Seidenraupen in der Lage sind, aus Kohlenhydraten im Organismus Fett zu bilden und abzulagern. Damit wird der Klärung des damals vielfach noch umstrittenen Problems der Fettbildung aus Kohlenhydraten im tierischen Organismus eine weitere Stütze gegeben und gleichzeitig gezeigt, daß diese Umwandlung auch bei niederen Organismen erfolgen kann.

Die Tätigkeit in Japan, für die ihm in Fachkreisen eine hohe Achtung und Anerkennung gezollt und die von der Regierung durch eine hohe Ordensauszeichnung geehrt wurde, fand ihren Abschluß durch die Berufung KELLNERS zum Direktor der Landwirtschaftlichen Versuchsstation Möckern als Nachfolger von Gustav KÜHN, der am 2. April 1892 im Alter von erst 52 Jahren an den Folgen einer Operation verstarb.

Gustav KÜHN, ein Schüler von Wilhelm HENNEBERG, hat die Versuchsstation Möckern seit 1867, also 25 Jahre, geleitet und das Arbeitsprofil der Versuchsstation in der Ausrichtung auf wissenschaftliche Forschungen auf dem Gebiet der Tierernährung maßgeblich geprägt. Für die weitere Entwicklung war entscheidend, daß KÜHN den Aufbau einer nach dem Pettenkoferschen Prinzip arbeitenden Respirationsapparatur für Ochsen 1881 abschließen und mit systematischen Untersuchungen zum Stoffumsatz, insbesondere durch Erfassung der N- und C-Bilanz, bei Wiederkäuern beginnen konnte. KÜHN war ein ausgezeichneter Analytiker, und er hat größten Wert auf Genauigkeit und Exaktheit bei wissenschaftlichen Arbeiten gelegt. Charakteristisch für ihn war, daß er nicht eher mit Forschungserbegnissen herauskam, bis er sie in Wiederholungen immer wieder bestätigt hatte. Die Wissenschaft soll nicht eher als Wegweiserin auftreten, ehe sie selbst den Weg gefunden hat. Das war die Richtschnur, die er seiner Arbeit gab und der er bis zum Lebensende treu geblieben ist. Die Genauigkeit seiner Arbeit mag dadurch gekennzeichnet werden, daß ein wissenschaftlich ausgebildeter Chemiker bei ihm erst 100 Übungsanalysen durchführen mußte, ehe er die gleiche Untersuchung in einem laufenden Versuch durchführen durfte.

Damit fand KELLNER, als er am 15. Februar 1893 die Leitung der Versuchsstation Möckern übernahm, experimentelle Bedingungen und gut geschulte Mitarbeiter vor, mit denen er seine Arbeiten, die ihm mit dem Aufbau seiner Stärkewertlehre weltweite Anerkennung erbracht haben, unverzüglich beginnen konnte. KELLNER hat mehrfach betont, welchen Nutzen er aus den Arbeiten KÜHNS für seine eigenen ziehen konnte. Und so betrachtete er es als seine erste Aufgabe, den wissenschaftlichen Nachlaß Gustav KÜHNS zu sichten, zu ordnen und bereits nach einem Jahr in einem umfangreichen Band der Zeitschrift „Die landwirtschaftlichen Versuchsstationen" zu veröffentlichen.

Als wesentliche Erweiterung der von KÜHN eingeführten Meßtechnik hat KELLNER – in logischer Konsequenz seiner erwähnten Gedankengänge aus dem Jahre 1880 – nach Einführung der Kalorimetrie in das Untersuchungsspektrum neben der stofflichen Bilanz (N- und C-Bilanzen) die energetische Bilanz bei den Arbeiten mit der Respirationstechnik einbezogen, eine Leistung, die wir vielleicht erst heute richtig würdigen können.

Den Schwerpunkt der Arbeiten in Möckern legte KELLNER auf die Erforschung des Stoff- und Energieumsatzes ausgewachsener Ochsen, um die energetische Wirkung der Hauptnährstoffe und repräsentativer Futtermittel unter definierten Bedingungen messen zu können. Er begann mit Untersuchungen zum Erhaltungsbedarf, schloß Untersuchungen über die Verwertung reiner isolierter Nährstoffe, die einer

Grundration in angemessener Höhe zugelegt wurde, an und führte dann Untersuchungen nach der Differenzmethodik mit einer Auswahl von Futtermitteln aus verschiedenen Futtermittelgruppen durch. Insgesamt hat KELLNER im Zeitraum von 1894–1911

149 Respirationsversuche mit ausgewachsenen Ochsen und
26 " " Milchkühen

durchgeführt.

KELLNER hat nur einen kleinen Teil seiner Versuche, und zwar 44, ausführlich veröffentlicht. Die Ergebnisse der anderen Versuche verwertete er in seinem Lehrbuch „Die Ernährung landwirtschaftlicher Nutztiere“ (1. Auflage: Parey-Verlag Berlin, 1905). Die Veröffentlichung der weiteren Materialien erfolgte zu etwa 30 % von Gustav FINGERLING, seinem Amtsnachfolger in Möckern, und 1953–55 von NEHRING und SCHIEMANN im Rahmen der Festschrift anläßlich des 100jährigen Bestehens der Landwirtschaftlichen Versuchsstation Leipzig-Möckern (Wiss. Abhandl., Dt. Akad. Landwirtsch.-Wiss., Berlin, Bd. V/1 (1953), Bd. V/2 (1954), Bd. V/3 (1956)).

Ich hatte das große Glück, den wissenschaftlichen Nachlaß Oskar KELLNERS bezüglich seiner Arbeiten mit der Respirationsversuchstechnik sichten und aufarbeiten zu dürfen.

Mich hat tief beeindruckt, mit welcher Konsequenz und Umsicht KELLNER die Experimente geleitet und ausgewertet hat. Seine erste Forderung war die nach äußerster Exaktheit in der experimentellen Durchführung der Versuche und der Protokollierung der Daten. Bestechend ist die klare Interpretation der Ergebnisse, wobei aus den umfangreich vorliegenden Handschriften die besondere Fähigkeit KELLNERS zur Niederschrift wissenschaftlicher und allgemeinverständlicher Publikationen ersichtlich ist, denn die Manuskripte enthalten kaum Korrekturen. Wurden Arbeiten KELLNERS angegriffen, so verstand er es vortrefflich, diese zu verteidigen, wobei er dann eine sehr spitze Feder führte. F. HONCAMP, einer seiner engeren Mitarbeiter und Schüler, drückte dies so aus: „KELLNER schrieb eine spröde Feder. Eine leichtfertige Kritik oder eine Entgegnung ohne genügendes Beweismaterial wurde fast immer in einer solchen Form zurückgewiesen, daß dem Betreffenden die Lust zu weiteren Angriffen gründlich vergangen war.“

Zutiefst beeindruckt hat mich ferner die Grundeinstellung KELLNERS zur Forschungstätigkeit an sich, die sehr modern anmutet; er postulierte, daß die Forschung auf dem von ihm gewählten Fachgebiet nicht Selbstzweck sein darf, sondern der Praxis dient. Sie muß von tiefgründigen, den naturwissenschaftlichen Erkenntnisstand voll ausschöpfenden Experimenten ausgehen. Die Ergebnisse dieser Experimente sind, sobald es der Forscher verantworten kann, entsprechend aufbereitet für die Praxis nutzbar zu machen. Diese Grundhaltung KELLNERS läßt sich sehr gut aus den folgenden Zitaten des in erster Auflage im Jahre 1905 erschienenen Lehrbuches „Die Ernährung der landwirtschaftlichen Nutztiere“ erkennen, die gleichzeitig seine Beweggründe für die Formung der Stärkewertlehre zum Ausdruck bringen.

So schreibt KELLNER im Vorwort der ersten Auflage seines Lehrbuches:

„Zu einer Zusammenfassung des bisher Erreichten erscheint der gegenwärtige Zeitpunkt besonders geeignet. Es ist durch die Untersuchungen des Verfassers über die Verwertung der einzelnen Nährstoffe und ganzer Futtermittel eine weitere Stufe in unserer Kenntnis der Vorgänge im Tierkörper erreicht und erkannt worden, daß die Futterzumessung nach verdaulichen Nährstoffen auf unrichtigen Voraussetzungen beruht. Der Gehalt der Futtermittel an verdaulichem Material deckt sich nicht mit ihrer Nährwirkung, vielmehr spielen hier der Verarbeitungsaufwand, die Fäulnis- und Zersetzungsvorgänge im Futterbrei und andere Dinge eine nicht zu unterschätzende Rolle. Die Untersuchung dieser Verhältnisse bei den hauptsächlichsten Vertretern der verschiedenen Futtermittelgruppen hat den Verfasser in den Stand gesetzt, die Wertschätzung der Futterstoffe und die Futterberechnung nunmehr auf die im Tiere selbst ermittelten Produktionswirkungen zu gründen. Das vorliegende Buch verläßt daher das bisher befolgte schablonenmäße Verfahren, die verdaulichen Nährstoffe zur alleinigen Grundlage zu nehmen und geht dazu über, die Eigenart jedes Futtermittels näher festzulegen und mit denjenigen Werten zu rechnen, von welchen die tierischen Leistungen abhängen. Manche Lücken, die noch der Ausfüllung harren, dürfen uns nicht davon abhalten, den als richtig erkannten Weg wirklich zu betreten; ist die Zahl der auf ihre Leistung untersuchten Futtermittel auch noch keine sehr große, so erreicht sie doch bereits annähernd denselben Stand, bei welchem man vormals die Rechnung mit Rohnährstoffen aufgab und das Futter nach seinem Gehalte an verdaulichen Nährstoffen zu bemessen anfing. Der neue Weg ist bereits soweit gangbar und sicher, daß er der Praxis geöffnet werden kann.

Neben dem Stoffumsatz, welcher bisher allein in der landwirtschaftlichen Fütterungslehre Berücksichtigung gefunden hat, sucht das vorliegende Lehrbuch auch die Verhältnisse des Energieumsatzes allenthalben zur Klärung der Vorgänge im Tierkörper heranzuziehen. Vieles, was bei der bisherigen einseitigen Behandlung der Tatsachen — bei der ausschließlichen Betrachtung des Stoffwechsels — unklar und undurchsichtig geblieben ist, wird durch die Betrachtung des Kraftwechsels dem Verständnis erheblich näher gerückt; ja die Fortschritte, welche in letzter Zeit auf dem Gebiet der Ernährungslehre gemacht worden sind, beruhen großenteils auf der Erforschung der energetischen Verhältnisse, die bei der Verwertung der Nahrung eine Rolle spielen".

Zur Einführung des Stärkewertes als Maßstab der energetischen Futterbewertung schreibt KELLNER in seinem Lehrbuch:

„Es fragt sich nun, wie man die produktive Wirkung eines Futtermittels oder einer Ration am zweckmäßigsten ausdrücken soll. Man könnte hier verschiedene Wege einschlagen und 1. den Ansatz, welchen das betreffende Futter, über den Erhaltungsbedarf hinaus gereicht, zu bewirken vermag, in Wärmemeßwerten angeben, das aber wenig geläufig ist und unnötig hohe Zahlen in die Berechnung hineinträgt. Man könnte 2. diesen Ansatz (Fett und Fleisch) auf Körperfett umrechnen und die so gewonnenen Zahlen benützen, aber auch dieses Verfahren erscheint insofern wenig geeignet, als es zu Mißdeutungen Veranlassung geben und bei manchen die Meinung wecken könnte, es käme überall und immer nur auf die Fetterzeugung an. Man kann 3. die gesamte energetische Wirkung eines Futtermittels so ausdrücken, als ob nur ein einziger vollwertiger Nährstoff zum Verzehr gebracht würde, und dieser Weg erscheint dem Verfasser als der gangbarste, obwohl er im Grunde genommen mit den beiden anderen Ausdrucksweisen dem Sinne nach identisch ist. Am geeignetsten, weil von dem bisher geübten Verfahren am wenigsten verschieden, ist es zweifellos, die in Rede stehende Wirkung so umzurechnen, als ob der wirksame Teil des Futters nur aus Stärkemehl bestände. Dieses Verfahren, die Rechnung mit Stärkewerten, wollen wir befolgen, dabei aber nicht außer acht lassen, daß dem verdaulichen Eiweiß besondere Funktionen zukommen, die von anderen Nährstoffen nicht geleistet werden können. Demzufolge werden wir überall außer dem Stärkewert, welcher sämtliche verdauliche Nährstoffe einschließt, noch die Menge des darin enthaltenen Eiweißes angeben."

Ganz modern mutet weiterhin an, daß KELLNER bereits Anfang unseres Jahrhunderts eine Reihe von Gemeinschaftsuntersuchungen zum rationellen Futtereinsatz unter Beteiligung verschiedener wissenschaftlicher Einrichtungen und von Praxisbetrieben nach einheitlichen Versuchsplänen organisierte. Auch hier möchte ich KELLNER zitieren, um seine progressive Denkweise, sein Verantwortungsbewußtsein als Wissenschaftler für die gesellschaftliche Entwicklung zu kennzeichnen. Bei Veröffentlichung des ersten Versuchsberichtes derartiger Gemeinschaftsversuche schrieb er:

„Wie auch die Versuche ausfallen würden, so würden die Ergebnisse für die fernere Gestaltung des Zusammenwirkens zwischen Praxis und Wissenschaft von Gewinn sein; sie würden ein schlagendes Beispiel für die Notwendigkeit der empfohlenen Einrichtungen bilden, insofern als sie eindringlich lehren werden, das Laboratoriumsexperimente nicht ohne weiteres auf die Praxis übertragen werden dürfen. Die deutsche Landwirtschaft hat genug Lehr- und Strafgeld dafür bezahlt, daß ihr bis jetzt nicht Gelegenheit geboten worden war, den Weg zu beschreiten, der eingeschlagen werden muß".

Insgesamt sind nach Plänen KELLNERS 5 große Versuchsreihen mit Milchkühen, Schweinen und Pferden durchgeführt worden, deren Ergebnisse von ihm bearbeitet und in den „Berichten über Landwirtschaft" veröffentlicht wurden.

KELLNER hat es trotz seines relativ frühen Todes miterleben können, daß seine Arbeit weltweit wissenschaftliche Anerkennung fand und sein Lebenswerk eine breite praktische Nutzanwendung erfuhr. So erschien sein Lehrbuch „Die Ernährung landwirtschaftlicher Nutztiere" bis zu seinem Tode in 5 Auflagen. Seine mehr populärwissenschaftliche Fassung „Grundzüge der Fütterungslehre" hatte bis dahin 3 Auflagen und wurde in 12 Sprachen übersetzt. Neben dieser wichtigen Publikationstätigkeit hat KELLNER bis zum Jahre 1910 „Biedermanns Centralblatt für Agrikulturchemie" und bis zu seinem Tode die Zeitschrift „Die landwirtschaftlichen Versuchsstationen" redigiert und maßgeblich mitgeprägt. Auf eine Fülle weiterer Aufgaben in der Leitung von Kommissionen, Ausschüssen usw., die ihn jedoch niemals von der Leitung der experimentellen Arbeit abhielten, möchte ich nicht weiter eingehen. Es ist mir kaum vorstellbar, wie er die riesige Arbeitslast bewältigen konnte, wobei ihm seine Schüler bescheinigen, daß er die Fülle an Arbeit in einer musterhaften Weise und mit einer unbedingten Zuverlässigkeit und Pünktlichkeit erledigte, wozu ihm sein klarer, scharfer Verstand, sein nie versagendes Gedächtnis, sein Bienenfleiß und seine rastlose Energie und Tatkraft verhalfen. KELLNERS Verdienste wurden vielfach geehrt, so mit der Verleihung des Titels „Geheimer Hofrat", zahlreichen hohen in- und ausländischen Orden, die erwähnte Ernennung zum Ehrendoktor der medizinischen Fakultät der Universität Breslau, die Verleihung der goldenen Liebig-Medaille, die Berufung zum Mitglied und Ehrenmitglied in einer Reihe von wissenschaftlichen Gesellschaften und landwirtschaftlichen Vereinen. Besonders hat er sich über die Ehrendoktorwürde und die Liebig-Medaille persönlich gefreut.

Abschließend möchte ich mich beim Vorstand der Sektion Tierernährung bedanken, daß ich zum Gedenken an Oskar KELLNER, der für mich einer meiner wissenschaftlichen Lehrer und ein unerreichbares Vorbild geworden ist, hier sprechen durfte. Wenn Sie gelegentlich in Leipzig sind und eine besinnliche Stunde finden, können Sie auf dem Südfriedhof in Leipzig, der in der Nähe des Völkerschlachtdenkmals liegt, die Grabstätte KELLNERS besuchen.

Der Grabstein trägt folgende Inschrift:

GEH. HOFRAT
Prof. Dr. Dr. h. c.
OSKAR KELLNER
13. 5. 1851–22. 9. 1911

EINER DER BEDEUTENDSTEN
DEUTSCHEN
TIERERNÄHRUNGSWISSENSCHAFTLER
UND BEGRÜNDER DER
WISSENSCHAFTLICHEN
FUTTERBEWERTUNG

Sektion Tierproduktion und Veterinärmedizin der Humboldt-Universität zu Berlin,
Bereich Tierernährung

O. SIMON

Untersuchungen zum Proteinumsatz beim Monogastriden*

Für jedermann leicht erfaßbare Größen in der Tierproduktion sind die tägliche Lebendmassezunahme und der Proteinansatz. Das Verständnis der Dinge wird komplizierter, wenn man sich vergegenwärtigt, daß der Proteinansatz lediglich die Differenz zwischen Proteinsyntheserate und Proteinabbaurate ist und daß die Proteinsyntheserate die Proteinansatzrate des Organismus stets um ein Mehrfaches übersteigt. Demnach ist der Proteinansatz das Ergebnis eines intensiven Proteinumsatzes.

Beim wachsenden Tier ist eine bestimmte Proteinansatzrate einerseits nicht zwangsläufig an eine bestimmte Proteinsyntheserate gebunden und andererseits kann die Proteinansatzrate sowohl durch Veränderungen in der Synthese – als auch der Abbaurate beeinflußt werden. So stellt das Verhältnis von angesetztem zu synthetisiertem Protein (auch als Effektivität der Proteinsynthese bezeichnet) keine konstante Größe dar.

Im Erhaltungszustand findet kein Proteinansatz statt, Synthese- und Abbaurate für die Proteine sind gleich groß. Aber auch in dieser Stoffwechselsituation kann der Proteinumsatz auf unterschiedlichem Niveau ablaufen. Solche Unterschiede könnten sich z. B. auf Messungen des Erhaltungsenergieumsatzes auswirken.

All dies verdeutlicht die Bedeutung der quantitativen Messung der Teilprozesse des Proteinumsatzes.

Um den Proteinumsatz näher zu charakterisieren, ist es erforderlich, zwei der drei Parameter Syntheserate, Abbaurate und Ansatzrate quantitativ zu bestimmen.

Während es kaum Methoden zur quantitativen Messung der Proteinabbaurate gibt, sind verschiedene Methoden zur Messung der Proteinsyntheserate im Gesamtorganismus oder in einzelnen Geweben entwickelt worden. Sie erfordern den Einsatz von mit Isotopen (^{14}C, ^{3}H, ^{35}S oder ^{15}N) markierten Aminosäuren und basieren auf verschiedenen mathematischen Modellen.

Alle Modelle stellen eine Vereinfachung der sehr komplizierten und vielfältigen Prozesse des Proteinumsatzes dar und beinhalten zahlreiche Annahmen, die den Kalkulationen zugrundegelegt werden. Diese Annahmen sind z. T. nur grobe Näherungen und müssen bei der Auswahl der Methodik zur Bearbeitung eines Problems kritisch analysiert und bei der Interpretation der Ergebnisse berücksichtigt werden.

Eigene Untersuchungen, die an Schweinen und Ratten mit ^{14}C-Aminosäuren durchgeführt wurden, sowie Untersuchungen anderer Arbeitsgruppen haben zu folgenden wesentlichen Ergebnissen geführt:

- Die fraktionelle Proteinsyntheserate ist in den einzelnen Organen sehr unterschiedlich. Sie liegt in Leber, Pankreas und Geweben des Verdauungstraktes um eine Zehnerpotenz höher als in der Skelettmuskulatur. In der Muskulatur von 30–60 kg schweren, wachsenden Schweinen beträgt der Wert 2,5–5,0 % des Eiweißbestandes der Muskulatur pro Tag.

* Vortrag anläßlich der Auszeichnung mit dem Arthur-Scheunert-Preis der Gesellschaft für Ernährung in der DDR am 1. 10. 1986

- Obwohl die Skelettmuskulatur etwa die Hälfte des Proteinbestandes des Organismus enthält, leistet sie lediglich nur 20–30 % der Proteinsynthese des Gesamtorganismus. Etwa die gleiche Syntheseleistung wird von den Geweben des Verdauungstraktes erbracht, die aber nur 6 % der Körperproteine enthalten. Diese Verhältnisse treffen auf alle untersuchten Tierarten zu.
- Für das intensiv wachsende Schwein kann abgeschätzt werden, daß die pro Zeiteinheit synthetisierte Proteinmenge ungefähr 5mal höher ist als die angesetzte Proteinmenge.
- Die Proteinsyntheserate unterliegt tagesrhythmischen Schwankungen, wobei es besonders in der Leber während der Resorptionsphase zur Stimulierung der Synthese kommt.
- Zahlreiche Parameter beeinflussen den Proteinumsatz. Dazu gehören u. a. genetische Herkunft, nutritive Faktoren, Alter und hormoneller Status.

Die intensiven Bemühungen zur Messung von Größen des Proteinumsatzes haben in den letzten Jahren zu einem nennenswerten Erkenntniszuwachs geführt. Dennoch sind quantitative Präzisierungen erforderlich und es sind zahlreiche Stoffwechselsituationen noch nicht ausreichend charakterisiert. Ein wesentlicher Grund hierfür ist, daß die zur Verfügung stehenden Techniken noch nicht empfindlich genug sind, um auch kleinere Differenzen in der Proteinsyntheserate zu bestimmen und daß es bisher noch überhaupt keine akzeptable Methode zur quantitativen Messung der Proteinabbaurate in vivo gibt.

So muß auch in Zukunft entscheidend an der Verbesserung der vorhandenen Techniken gearbeitet werden.

Forschungszentum für Tierproduktion Dummerstorf-Rostock
der Akademie der Landwirtschaftswissenschaften der DDR,
Bereich Tierernährung „Oskar Kellner“

L. Schmidt, F. Weissbach und H.-J. Block

Wissenschaftliche Grundlagen und technologische Möglichkeiten für den chemischen Aufschluß von Getreidestroh mit Ammoniak

Eine Möglichkeit des Strohaufschlusses ist die Behandlung von feuchtem Stroh mit Ammoniak bzw. mit Harnstoff als Ammoniakquelle, durch die das Stroh konserviert, aufgeschlossen und mit NPN angereichert wird. Die Verwendung von Harnstoff anstelle von wasserfreiem Ammoniak oder Ammoniakwasser ist aus technologischen Gründen und in bezug auf den Arbeits- und Gesundheitsschutz vorteilhaft. In feuchtem Stroh erfolgt bei ausreichendem Wassergehalt sowohl unter aeroben als auch unter anaeroben Lagerungsbedingungen spontan eine kontinuierliche Hydrolyse des Harnstoffes zu NH_3 und CO_2; und zwar über die Zwischenstufen Ammoniumkarbamat und Ammoniumkarbonat. Die dazu erforderliche Urease wird von im Stroh vorhandenen Mikroorganismen gebildet. Ammoniak ist die wirksame Substanz, sowohl für die Konservierung gegen den aeroben (Schimmelbildung) und anaeroben (Buttersäurebildung) Verderb als auch für den verdaulichkeitsverbessernden Aufschluß, die beide im alkalischen Bereich (pH 7–9) erfolgen.

Das Verfahrensprinzip wird bisher bei der Konservierung von Quadergroßballen aus feuchtem Stroh (Verfahrensentwicklung vom FZM Schlieben/Bornim) und bei der silageähnlichen Lagerung von feuchtem Häckselstroh in Horizontal- und Hochsilos genutzt.

Die Harnstoffhydrolyse und damit die Anreicherung von NH_3 sowie die Erhöhung des pH-Wertes setzen in Abhängigkeit von der Strohfeuchte schnell ein. Bereits nach 1tägiger Lagerung in Silos sind bei 40 % Strohfeuchte etwa 70 % des zugesetzten Harnstoffes hydrolysiert. Das Ausmaß des Aufschlußeffektes wird vor allem von der Strohfeuchte, der Harnstoffdosis und der Lagerungstemperatur beeinflußt. Gezielte Modellversuche in thermostatisierten Behältern führten zu dem Ergebnis, daß 50 % Strohfeuchte, eine Harnstoffdosis von 8 % (bezogen auf TS) und 50–60 °C Lagerungstemperatur optimale Bedingungen für den Strohaufschluß sind.

Unter diesen Bedingungen kann der Aufschlußprozeß schon nach 2wöchiger Lagerungsdauer abgeschlossen sein.

Die Lagerungstemperatur hat bei ausreichender Strohfeuchte, NH_3-Konzentration und Lagerungsdauer einen entscheidenden Einfluß auf die Aufschlußintensität.

Die Auswertung von Produktionsexperimenten ergab, daß bei silageähnlicher Lagerung von harnstoffbehandeltem feuchtem Häckselstroh Aufschlußeffekte von durchschnittlich 14 Verdaulichkeitseinheiten, entsprechend etwa 100 EFr/kg TS zu erwarten sind. Bei der Harnstoffbehandlung von feuchtem Quadergroßballenstroh wurden infolge niedrigerer Strohfeuchten durchschnittlich nur Futterwerterhöhungen um 8 Verdaulichkeitseinheiten, entsprechend 60 EFr/kg TS ermittelt.

Sektion Tierproduktion und Veterinärmedizin der Karl-Marx-Universität Leipzig, Wissenschaftsbereich Tierernährungschemie, Jena

G. Flachowsky

Physikalische, chemische und biologische Methoden der Strohaufbereitung und Möglichkeiten der praktischen Anwendung

Die Beurteilung des Behandlungseffektes von Stroh sollte neben Test- (in vitro, in sacco) und Verdauungsversuchen vor allem durch langfristige Fütterungsversuche erfolgen.

In der nachfolgenden tabellarischen Darstellung wird der Einfluß verschiedener Behandlungen von Weizenstroh auf die in vivo-Verdaulichkeit (Mittel aus 3 bis 5 Verdauungsversuchen an je 5 Hammeln) und die relative Stroh- und Energieaufnahme sowie Lebendmassezunahme von Mastbullen (Mittel von 9 Einzelfütterungsversuchen, Fütterung: 2 kg Konzentrat/Tier und Tag, Stroh ad lib., Häckselstroh = 100 %) wiedergegeben.

Strohbehandlung	Verdaulichkeit der organischen Substanz (%)	Relative Strohaufnahme		Relative Lebendmassezunahme
		Trockensubstanz	Nettoenergie	
gehäckselt	45	100 (3,4 kg/Tag)	100 (1,1 kEFr/Tag)	100 (476 g/Tag)
grob gemahlen	45	107	106	96
gemahlen, pelletiert	43	138	136	121
gehäckselt, mit 2,5 % NH_3 behandelt	53	119	148	154
gehäckselt, feucht mit 4 % Harnstoff behandelt	53	145	168	153
gehäckselt, mit Schafharn behandelt (Stroh : Harn = 1 : 2)	52	95*	111*	
gehäckselt, mit 5 % NaOH besprüht	59	118	153	135
defibrilliert, mit 4 % NaOH behandelt	58	130	166	153
gemahlen, bei Pelletierung mit 2 % NaOH behandelt	59	192	244	188

* Versuche mit Schafen

Sektion Tierproduktion und Veterinärmedizin der Humboldt-Universität zu Berlin, Bereich Tierernährung[1], LPG (T) Schauen, Krs. Halberstadt[2]

H. BERGNER[1], R. GÖRSCH[1], B. BETZIN[1], J. MARIENBURG[1] und H. LUBINETZKI[2]

NH_3-Strohaufschluß bei einer NH_3-Entwicklung aus Harnstoff-Kohlenhydratmischungen

Es ist bekannt, daß NH_3 aus Harnstoff mit Hilfe mikrobieller Urease entwickelt werden kann und im Falle einer Harnstoffzugabe (H) zu feuchtem Stroh sowohl eine konservierende Wirkung als auch eine Aufschlußwirkung eintritt. Voraussetzung ist es hierbei, daß ein möglichst guter Luftabschluß unter den Bedingungen einer silageähnlichen Lagerung bei hohem Wassergehalt (mehr als 50 %) gewährleistet wird, um die Entwicklung der aeroben Pilze (Verschimmeln des Strohs) zu unterdrücken. Unseren Untersuchungen lag der Gedanke zugrunde, durch eine Beimischung von leichtlöslichen Kohlenhydraten zum Harnstoff die bakterielle Ureasebildung so zu stimulieren, daß die raschere NH_3-Freisetzung ausreicht, um auf aufwendigen Siloraum verzichten zu können, die Wasserzugabe zu verringern und ein ganzjährig anwendbares Verfahren für den NH_3-Strohaufschluß zu entwickeln.

Wir prüften unter Laborbedingungen Mischungen aus Zucker (Saccharose, Z) und Harnstoff (H), die einer Strohmehlmenge von etwa 350 g zugesetzt und in Plastetüten gelagert wurden.

Der Wassergehalt der Strohmischung wurde auf 20, 30 und 40 % begrenzt und in die zu gleichen Teilen gemischten Zucker-Harnstoffmengen auf 6, 8 bzw. 10 % (bezogen auf die Stroh-TS) hinzugefügt. Für die NH_3-Freisetzung ergaben sich die höchsten Werte bei 10 % ZH. Obwohl infolge der geringen Mengen keine deutlichen Temperatursteigerungen nachweisbar waren, gab es mit steigendem Wassergehalt nicht nur eine Verdreifachung (20 % → 40 % Wasser) der NH_3-Freisetzung, sondern auch eine drastische Verkürzung des NH_3-Maximums (20 % H_2O nach 23 d, 30 % H_2O nach 9 d, 40 % H_2O nach 3 d). Der Unterschied hinsichtlich des absoluten NH_3-Maximums zwischen der ZH-Variante und 5 % H alleine blieb jedoch in allen H_2O-Varianten zugunsten von ZH bestehen. Wurden die Strohproben (mit 30 % H_2O) im Brutschrank (37 °C) gelagert, so waren bereits nach 24 h Lagerung in der ZH-Variante noch 46 % und in der H-Variante 66 % des H nachweisbar. Der zugesetzte Zucker wird von den Mikroorganismen genutzt, jedoch zu anderen Metaboliten (z. B. Milchsäure) umgesetzt. Bei Markierung von Z mittels ^{14}C-Saccharose wurde in der Variante „10 % ZH, 30 % H_2O" in 8 Tagen nur 1 % der Radioaktivität als $^{14}CO_2$ nachgewiesen, und 90 % der Radioaktivität konnten aus der Strohmischung heiß ausgewaschen werden.

In der LPG (T) Schauen, Krs. Halberstadt wurden Mischungen aus Stroh, 6 % H + 18 % Melasse und 6 % Dextrose an 223 Mastbullen im Lebendmasseabschnitt von 256 bis 507 kg verfüttert. Die höhere TS-Aufnahme aus reinem Stroh betrug 1,3 kg in der Versuchsgruppe im Gegensatz zu den 241 Kontrolltieren, die im Durchschnitt nur 1,1 kg Stroh-TS/Tier · Tag verzehrten. Die durchschnittlich höhere Tageszunahme in Höhe von 177 g in der Versuchsgruppe (715 g/Tier · d) resultiert aus dem Mehrverzehr von 1,3 kg Aufschlußstroh + 0,45 kg Melasse + Dextrose, wobei etwa 130 g tägliche Mehrzunahme dem NH_3-Aufschlußeffekt und dem höheren Strohverzehr zuzurechnen sind.

Die sehr rasche NH_3-Freisetzung bei Zugabe von leichtlöslichen Kohlenhydraten zum Stroh erfordert unter Praxisbedingungen keinen Luftabschluß und ermöglicht einen relativ hohen TS-Gehalt (60 %). Ohne Abdeckung ist das Endprodukt nicht lagerfähig; jedoch ist eine NH_3-Einwirkungszeit von etwa 5–7 Tagen zur Verbesserung des Aufschlußeffektes zweckmäßig.

Sektion Tierproduktion und Veterinärmedizin der Karl-Marx-Universität Leipzig, Wissenschaftsbereich Tierernährungschemie, Jena[1]
Lehr- und Versuchsstation Remroda[2]

M. SCHNEIDER[1], G. CYRIACI[2], G. RICHTER[1] und G. FLACHOWSKY[1]

Untersuchungen zum Futterwert von NH_3-begastem Weizenstroh

Anhand einer umfangreichen Literaturauswertung konnte gezeigt werden, daß die NH_3-Begasung von Stroh zu einer höheren Verdaulichkeit und gesteigerter Strohaufnahme führt.

In 10 Verdauungsversuchen mit Hammeln bzw. SMR-Mastbullen (300 kg) sowie 3 Einzelfütterungsversuchen mit SMR-Mastbullen (Anfangsmasse 193 bis 225 kg) zu verschiedenen Problemstellungen (Vergleich unbehandeltes und NH_3-begastes Stroh,

Vergleich zweier NH_3-Stroh-Chargen mit unterschiedlichem Aufschlußgrad, verschieden hohe Konzentratgaben) wurde der Einfluß der NH_3-Begasung unter den in der DDR üblichen Srohlagerungsvarianten hinsichtlich der Beeinflussung des Futterwertes von Weizenstroh geprüft.

Die Verdaulichkeit der organischen Substanz stieg durch NH_3-Begasung im Mittel der Verdauungsversuche um 11 Einheiten an. Gegenüber unbehandeltem Stroh nahmen Bullen bei gleichem Strohverzehr (2 kg Konzentrat je Tier und Tag) 106 g je Tag mehr zu, wenn das Stroh mit NH_3 begast war. Bei ad libitum Aufnahme betrug der Mehrverzehr an NH_3-Stroh etwa 0,7 kg pro Tier und Tag, die Bullen nahmen täglich 161 g mehr zu.

Der Aufschlußeffekt nach NH_3-Begasung war bei feuchtem Stroh (80,3 gegenüber 87,3 % TS) größer und äußerte sich in höherer Strohaufnahme und etwa 250 g Mehrzunahme je Tier und Tag, wenn neben 2 kg Konzentrat NH_3-Stroh ad libitum gefüttert wurde. Unter bestimmten Bedingungen kann NH_3-begastes Stroh als Hauptgrobfutterquelle eingesetzt werden (Tiere mit niedrigem Leistungsniveau), wo es den Energieerhaltungsbedarf abdeckt. In einem Testversuch (112 Tage) konnte bei alleiniger Verabreichung von NH_3-Stroh eine mittlere Tageszunahme von 413 g erzielt werden.

Forschungszentrum für Tierproduktion Dummerstorf-Rostock der Akademie der Landwirtschaftswissenschaften der DDR, Bereich Tierernährung „Oskar Kellner"

W. Jentsch

Energieansatz bei Verfütterung von Aufschlußstroh im Gesamtstoffwechselversuch

In 40 Gesamtstoffwechselversuchen an 8 ausgewachsenen Hammeln wurde der Einfluß der Langzeitlagerung (1 1/2 und 2 1/2 Jahre) von Feuchtstroh (durchschnittlich 40 % Wassergehalt) im Vergleich zu unbehandeltem Winterroggenstroh in Rationen mit 2/3 Stroh und 1/3 Gerstenschrot auf Verdaulichkeit und Energieumsatz geprüft. Langzeitlagerung von Feuchtstroh mit Harnstoffzusatz führt zu einer Erhöhung der Verdaulichkeit der Energie bzw. der organ. Substanz um 12–15 Verdaulichkeitseinheiten, die durch eine Verbesserung der Verdaulichkeit der Rohkohlenhydrate bedingt ist. Der in der Erhöhung der Verdaulichkeit nachzuweisende Aufschlußeffekt bleibt nach Energieumsatzmessungen mittels Respirationsversuchstechnik bis zum Energieansatz wirksam.

Gemessene Energiekennzahlen der Rationen in MJ/kg TS

Strohgaben in g/Tier · d	Trockenstroh 615	Harnstoffeuchtstroh 568	553	689
Bruttoenergie	18,88	18,73	18,96	18,98
Verdauliche Energie	9,58	10,99	11,03	11,03
umsetzbare Energie	8,30	9,43	9,28	9,33
Energie für Erhaltung und Ansatz	3,70	4,95	4,62	4,82

Die im DDR-Futterbewertungssystem gegebenen Grundlagen der energetischen Bewertung der Futtermittel sind auch für chemisch behandeltes Stroh anzuwenden.

Die Erhöhung der Energiekonzentration des Winterroggenstrohs von etwa 300 auf 400 EFr/kg TS ist z. Z. durch die Prinzipien der Futtermitteluntersuchung und -attestierung (gleicher Rohfasergehalt) nicht bestimmbar.

Sektion Tierproduktion und Veterinärmedizin der Karl-Marx Universität Leipzig, Wissenschaftsbereich Tierernährungschemie, Jena[1]
Zentralinstitut für Isotopen- und Strahlenforschung der Akademie der Wissenschaften der DDR, Leipzig[2]

M. SCHNEIDER[1], W. I. OCHRIMENKO[1], G. FLACHOWSKY[1], M. BÄR[2] und A. HENNIG[1]

Untersuchungen zur in sacco-Verdaulichkeit von unterschiedlich vorbehandeltem und anschließend bestrahltem Weizenstroh

Mit Hilfe der Nylonbeutel-Methode wurde der Trockensubstanzverlust nach 48 h Panseninkubation bei Hammeln von unterschiedlich vorbehandeltem und dann bestrahltem (γ-Strahlen) Weizenstroh bestimmt. Der durch die Bestrahlung hervorgerufene und die Vorbehandlung beeinflußte höhere TS-Verlust im Pansen ist zum größten Teil mit einem Anstieg der Auswaschung (Löslichkeitserhöhung, Partikelzerkleinerung) erklarbar. Der mikrobielle Abbau der nicht auswaschbaren Strohtrockensubstanz wurde in den Untersuchungen vorwiegend von der chemischen Vorbehandlung beeinflußt.

Im einzelnen ergaben sich für den Trockensubstanzverlust nach Panseninkubation folgende Werte:

Bestrahlungsdosis (MGy)		NaOH 2 %	NaOH 4 %	KOH 2 %	KOH 4 %	$Ca(OH)_2$ 2 %	$Ca(OH)_2$ 4 %	NaOH/KOH 2 %	NaOH/KOH 4 %	Kontrolle (H_2O)
0	$\bar{x}$	41,7[A,a]	60,5[b]	40,8[A,a]	49,1	32,1[c]	39,3[a]	45,6[A]	57,3[A,b]	30,5[A,c]
	s	3,0	3,1	2,1	1,6	2,6	2,1	2,2	2,0	0,8
0,1	$\bar{x}$	44,9[A,a]	66,1[A]	41,6[A,b]	54,6[A,c]	39,2[A]	43,3[A,a,b]	44,6[A,a]	58,8[A,c]	32,2[A,B]
	s	1,6	3,4	1,9	3,9	1,4	1,4	1,2	1,7	3,3
0,25	$\bar{x}$	49,0[a]	68,8[A,b]	41,4[A,c]	52,3[A]	41,0[A,c]	43,3[A,c]	49,7[a]	66,4[b]	35,4[B]
	s	1,2	2,0	2,7	1,7	2,4	1,4	1,5	2,7	1,6
0,5	$\bar{x}$	54,4[a]	78,2	48,0[b]	66,3	47,3[b]	54,5[a]	53,4[a]	70,9	40,0
	s	2,2	3,8	1,9	2,4	1,8	1,2	2,7	1,9	2,3
1,0	$\bar{x}$	71,2	92,0	60,0[a]	84,3	60,7[a]	65,7[b]	64,6[b]	77,3	53,2
	s	1,1	2,4	2,2	1,0	1,4	2,3	3,4	3,8	2,7

A, B Werte in einer Spalte mit gleichen Buchstaben sind nicht signifikant verschieden ($p<0,05$)
a, b, c Werte in einer Zeile mit gleichen Buchstaben sind nicht signifikant verschieden ($p<0,05$)

Sektion Tierproduktion und Veterinärmedizin der Humboldt-Universität zu Berlin, Bereich Tierfütterung und Ernährungsschäden

H. MÜNCHOW und M. FINGER

Möglichkeiten des Einsatzes verschieden behandelter Strohmaterialien in der Fütterung von Absetzferkeln – ein Beitrag zur Leistungsstabilisierung und Konzentrateinsparung

Aus unter experimentellen Versuchsbedingungen durchgeführten Untersuchungen mit Absetzferkeln unterschiedlichen Absetztermins (35., 42. und 49. Lebenstag) werden Ergebnisse vorgestellt, die die Einsatzwürdigkeit verschieden behandelter Strohmaterialien (HCl-Strohmehl = HCl-behandelt ohne Dämpfaufschluß, teilhydrolysiertes Strohmehl = HCl-behandelt mit nachfolgendem Dämpfaufschluß; beide Varianten jeweils ohne sowie mit Neutralisationsmittel zur Mischfutterherstellung verwendet) im Vergleich zur alleinigen Konzentratfütterung bzw. deren Kombination mit unbehandeltem Strohmehl sowie Weizenkleie unter Beweis stellen.

Als Bewertungskriterien dienten in diesem Zusammenhang die speziellen (Zunahme, Futter- und Energieaufwand) und allgemeinen Leistungen der Tiere (Gesundheitsstatus, Tierverluste) sowie Einflußgrößen auf die Nährstoffverdaulichkeit der Gesamtration und Faktoren zur diätetischen Wirkung der Rohfaserträger (Verzehrsbeeinflussung, Milieuveränderungen im Magen sowie im Dickdarmbereich, Beeinflussung des Verdauungsepithels u. a. m.).

Bei Integration von HCl-behandelten Strohmaterialien (etwa 10 % der Tr.-Subst. der Futtermischung) verbesserten sich die speziellen Leistungen um 8–20 %, wobei von den nicht neutralisierten HCl-Behandlungsvarianten der höhere Wirkungseffekt ausging.

Dieser wird im Zusammenhang mit einer physiologischen Doppelwirkung diskutiert (gut fermentierbare, hinsichtlich Schadmikroben unbedenkliche Rohfaserquelle sowie Futterkomponente mit geringer Pufferkapazität) und diesbezügliche Wirkungsprinzipien herausgestellt (Erhöhung der Energieaufnahme durch Verzehrsstimulierung positive Beeinflussung der Proteinverdaulichkeit, Senkung des Magen-pH-Wertes, Stimulierung der FFS-Produktion, verringerter Antigendruck, Gesunderhaltung des Darmepithels, Blutharnstoff- und Cholesterolgehalt senkende Wirkung u. a. m.).

Sektion Tierproduktion und Veterinärmedizin der Humboldt-Universität zu Berlin, Bereich Sozialistische Betriebswirtschaft

S. JAHN, H.-J. THIEME, E. WÜSTENHAGEN und R. SCHMIDT

Auswirkungen des Einsatzes von HCl-behandeltem Strohmehl auf das wirtschaftliche Ergebnis in der Ferkelproduktion – dargestellt an Produktionsversuchen

In der LPG Industrielle Schweinezucht Frankenförde erfolgt seit mehreren Jahren der Einsatz von behandeltem Strohmehl in der Ferkel- und Sauenfütterung. Eine betriebseigene Aufbereitungsanlage hat einen Strohdurchsatz von 30 dt je Schicht.

Die Herstellungskosten betragen 13,15 M je dt HCl-behandeltes Strohmehl und infolge eines zusätzlichen Dämpfprozesses 18,90 M je dt teilhydrolysiertes Strohmehl. Absatzferkel erhielten während der gesamten Gruppenaufzuchthaltung neben Konzentraten (Ferkelstarterfutter und Ferkelaufzuchtfutter) HCl-behandeltes Strohmehl mit einem Anteil von 10 %. Im absetznahen Zeitraum sanken Morbiditäts- und Mortalitätsrate. Die täglichen Lebendmassezunahmen lagen mit durchschnittlich 380 g je Tier und Tag um 4,5 % unter denen der Kontrolltiere. Jedoch sanken der Aufwand an Konzentratfuttermitteln um 8,3 % und an Futterenergie um 5,5 %. Parallel dazu konnten 6 % Futterkosten eingespart werden. Infolge der ganzzeitigen konzentratsparenden Fütterung in der Gruppenaufzuchthaltung reduzierte sich der Gewinn nur um 1,50 M je Jungschwein (35 kg Lebendmasse). Der Kostensatz erhöhte sich um 0,3 Einheiten.

Folgende futterökonomische Kennzahlen zur Produktion von Absetzferkeln unter Zusatz von behandeltem Strohmehl wurden erzielt:

	Maßeinheit	Kontrollgruppen		Versuchsgruppen (Stroh)*	
			relativ		relativ
Lebendmassezunahme	g/Tag	398	100,0	380	95,5
Konzentrataufwand	kg/kg LMZ	2,42	100,0	2,22	91,7
Energieaufwand	kEFs/kg LMZ	1,46	100,0	1,38	94,5
Futterkosten	M/kg LMZ	2,52	100,0	2,37	94,0
Gewinn	M/Tier	90,20	100,0	88,70	98,3
Kostensatz		75,10		75,40	

* Mit 10 % HCl-behandeltem Strohmehl als Zusatz

Sektion Tierproduktion und Veterinärmedizin der Karl-Marx-Universität Leipzig, Wissenschaftsbereich Tierernährungschemie, Jena

A. Hennig

Tierexkremente im Futtermittel

Schweinekot enthält ≈ 20 % Rohprotein in der Trockensubstanz, und seine organische Substanz wird beim Rind zu ≈ 52 % verdaut. Da Feststoffe aus Schweinegülle nicht lagerbeständig sind, setzten wir ihnen, bezogen auf 100 kg Trockensubstanz, 2 kg Harnstoff zu. Diese behandelten Feststoffe erwiesen sich über 2 Monate lagerfähig; durch die Behandlung mit Harnstoff konnte der Futterwert um 30–50 EFr/kg Trockensubstanz erhöht werden. Um die Hochpolymere der Feststoffe besser zu nutzen, behandelten wir die Feststoffe mit 2 kg NaOH/kg Trockensubstanz und erhöhten dadurch den Futterwert um weitere 50 EFr/kg TS. Höhere Laugenkonzentrationen verbesserten den Futterwert nicht linear. Äquimolare Mengen KOH erzeugten den gleichen Aufschlußeffekt im Vergleich zur NaOH. $Ca(OH)_2$ konnte die beiden anderen Alkalien zur Hälfte ohne Rückgang der Aufschlußwirkung ersetzen. Der Einsatz von $Ca(OH)_2$ und KOH als Aufschlußmittel hat in bezug auf Tiergesundheit und Bodenfruchtbarkeit Vorteile gegenüber NaOH.

In langfristigen Fütterungsversuchen mit Mastrindern zeigten wir, daß Güllefeststoffe bis 50 % des Energiebedarfes decken können, jedoch sind Einsatzmenge und Futteraufnahme vor allem vom Trockensubstanzgehalt der Schweinegüllefeststoffe abhängig. Die geringe Partikelgröße der Feststoffe erhöht die Aufenthaltsdauer im Pansen und verbessert deshalb die Futteraufnahme je kg Lebendmasse um 20–30 % gegenüber gebräuchlichen Maissilagerationen. Dieser hohe Verzehr erklart auch die guten Zunahmen, welche mit hohen Feststoffanteilen in der Ration bei 2 kg Konzentrat/Bulle und Tag erzielt wurden. Die Schlachtkörperqualität und Qualitat von Dauerwurst und Schinken wurden durch Feststoffe in der Ration der Mastbullen nicht negativ verändert.

Schweinegüllefeststoffe sind futterwürdig, wenn sie mit je 2 kg NaOH (s.o.) und Harnstoff behandelt werden. Die Kosten je kEFr sind billiger als bei jedem anderen Futtermittel. Feststoffe werden am besten mit anderen Grobfuttermitteln (Silage, Grünfutter) verfüttert; der Anteil der Feststoffe an der Rationstrockensubstanz der Mastrinder sollte in der Praxis 30 % betragen. Die geringe Partikelgroße der Feststoffe erfordert bei hoheren Anteilen in der Ration die Zufütterung von 1–2 kg Heu oder Stroh, da die Rohfaser der Feststoffe nur zu 1/6 im Vergleich zu Stroh pansenmotorisch wirksam ist.

Die Rezyklierung von Exkrementen der Nichtwiederkäuer an Nichtwiederkäuer ist nicht möglich, da bei der zweiten Passage nur noch wenig verdaut wird. In noch größerem Maße gilt das für die Verfütterung der Wiederkauerexkremente an Schweine und Geflügel. Ausnahmen würden gültig sein, wenn dieser Kot in geringen Mengen zur Beseitigung eines Vitamin-B_{12}-Defizits genutzt werden sollte. Wiederkäuerkot kann auch nach Behandlung mit Aufschlußmitteln nicht mit Nutzen an die gleiche Tierart verfüttert werden.

Broilertiefstreu ist nach 14tägiger Lagerung in überdachten Raumen in Abhangigkeit von der Einstreu ein wertvolles Futter für Mastrinder. Legehennenexkremente erfordern meist wegen ihres hohen H_2O-Gehaltes eine Trennung in Feststoffe und Fugat. Die sehr aschereichen Feststoffe werden im Gemisch mit Stroh und anderem Futter gut gefressen, aber ihre Einsatzmenge muß auf 0,5 kg TS/100 kg Lebendmasse bebegrenzt werden. Jeder Exkrementeinsatz bedarf in unserem Lande der Zustimmung des Kreistierarztes.

LPG „Das Volk", Aschara[1]
Sektion Tierproduktion und Veterinärmedizin der Karl-Marx-Universität Leipzig, Wissenschaftsbereich Tierernährungschemie, Jena[2]
Chemiekombinat Bitterfeld[3]

M. Bugdol[1], D. Wolfram[1], K.-H. Bodenstein[1], G. Flachowsky[2], A. Hennig[2] und G. Kreuzberger[3]

Vergleichende Prüfung von KOH- und NaOH-behandelten Schweinegüllefeststoffen auf Verdaulichkeit und Mastergebnisse bei Wiederkauern

In der LPG „Das Volk" Aschara wurden Güllefeststoffe mit NaOH oder KOH behandelt. Eine repräsentative Charge aus dem Bullenmastversuch V_2 wurde entnommen und mittels der Differenzmethode an Hammeln auf ihre Verdaulichkeit geprüft, folgende Resultate wurde erhalten:

Behandlung (bezogen auf TS)	Scheinbare Verdaulichkeit (%) organische Substanz	Rohkohlenhydrate
unbehandelt	28,9	31,5
2 % NaOH	44,8	46,8
2,8 % KOH	43,4	46,3

Es wurden 2 Fütterungsversuche über 273 (V_1) bzw. 263 (V_2) Tage an Mastbullen der Rasse SMR durchgeführt. Die Tiere standen in Anbindehaltung. 12 Tiere waren jeweils zu einer Gruppe zusammengefaßt. In beiden Versuchen erhielten die Tiere neben unterschiedlich behandelten Güllefeststoffen, ad libitum (NaOH- bzw. KOH-behandelte Feststoffe, Mischung NaOH-KOH-behandelte Feststoffe 1 : 1) 1,7 kg Konzentratmischung und 1 kg gehäckseltes Weizenstroh je Tier und Tag.

Mastergebnisse (V_1; 224 kg, V_2; 259 kg Anfangsmasse, je Tier)

Feststoffbehandlung (bezogen auf TS)	Versuch 1 1,3 % NaOH	1,5 % KOH	Mischg. 1 : 1	Versuch 2 2 % NaOH	2,8 % KOH	Mischg. 1 : 1
TS-Aufnahme (kg/Tier u. Tag)	9,0	9,0	9,1	9,6	9,9	9,9
Lebendmassezunahme (g/Tier u. Tag)	856	802	816	841	850	846
Energieaufwand (kEFr/kg Zunahme)	4,9	5,0	5,0	4,8	4,9	4,9

Zwischen den Gruppen beider Versuche waren die Unterschiede im Mastergebnis nur gering und nicht signifikant.

Sektion Tierproduktion und Veterinärmedizin der Karl-Marx-Universität Leipzig, Wissenschaftsbereich Tierernährungschemie, Jena

G. Richter, G. Flachowsky, K.-H. Bodenstein und D. Wolfram

Konzentratarme Fütterung von Mastbullen mit Schweinegüllefeststoff-Maissilage-Rationen

In einem Testversuch mit 8 Mastbullen (317 Versuchstage) und zwei Gruppenfütterungsversuchen mit 58 bzw. 114 Mastbullen (273 bzw. 168 Versuchstage) wurden Feststoff-Maissilage-Mischungen (Testversuch: 1 : 1; Versuche I und II: 1 : 1,5, auf Frischmassebasis) und unterschiedliche Konzentratmengen (Testversuch: 0; Versuche I und II: 0 : 1 bzw. 2 g Konzentratmischung je Tier und Tag) verabreicht. Im Versuch II wurde an eine Kontrollgruppe Maissilage ad libitum und 2 kg Konzentrat je Tier und Tag gefüttert. Im Testversuch und beiden Fütterungsversuchen verzehrten die Mastbullen ohne Konzentrateinsatz ≈2,5 kg TS/100 kg Lebendmasse und Tag, die Zunahmen betrugen 819, 797 bzw. 522 g/Tier und Tag. Durch Konzentratgaben stieg die Lebendmassezunahme an (Versuch I: 1 bzw. 2 kg/Tier und Tag: 912 bzw. 930; Versuch II: 1 bzw. 2 kg/Tier und Tag: 786 bzw. 872 g/Tier und Tag). Die Lebendmassezunahme der mit Maissilage-Konzentrat-Mischung gefütterten Bullen war annähernd mit der der Maissilage-Kontrollgruppe vergleichbar (872 bzw. 897 g/Tier und Tag).

Die Hauptursache für die unterschiedlichen Ergebnisse in den Versuchen I und II wird im Trockensubstanz- bzw. Energiegehalt von Feststoffen und Maissilage (Testversuch, Versuch I bzw. II, TS-Gehalt der Feststoffe: 46,4; 45,0 bzw. 40,1 %; TS-Gehalt der Maissilage: 27,8; 25,7 bzw. 20,3 %) gesehen.

Bei Bereitstellung trockensubstanz- (25–30 % TS) und energiereicher Maissilage (>560 EFr/kg TS) sind Feststoff-Maissilage-Mischungen (1 : 1 bis 2) ohne wesentliche Konzentratergänzung vor allem für die Vormast der Bullen geeignet, in der Endmast ist für höhere Zunahmen eine Konzentratergänzung zweckmäßig (2–3 kg/Tier und Tag).

LPG (T) Worin, Bezirk Frankfurt/O.

W. Schulze

Futterwert und Einsatzmöglichkeiten von Broilertiefstreu

In der LPG (T) Worin wird seit 1971 Broilertiefstreu (BT) mit Erfolg in der Rindermast (jährlich 1500–2000 t) bei Rationsanteilen von 1–4 kg je Tier und Tag eingesetzt. Damit werden mindestens 80 % des Rohproteinbedarfes der Mastbullen gedeckt.

Die Nutzung der insgesamt in der DDR anfallenden BT ist unzureichend und teilweise rückläufig. Zusammenfassung der im Rahmen der staatlichen Futtermittelprüfung erfaßten Analysenwerte (Information der Zentralstelle Halle-Lettin) zeigen in den letzten Jahren bei starken Schwankungen einen deutlichen Rückgang in der Energiekonzentration und gegenüber den Werten der Futtermitteltabellen einen Rückgang auf 80 %. Ursachen und Zusammenhänge werden diskutiert.

Die aus der LPG Broilermast Marxwalde in Worin zum Einsatz gekommene BT konnte im energetischen Futterwert stabil gehalten werden.

Für die Erhaltung eines möglichst hohen Futterwertes in der BTS werden folgende Maßnahmen für erforderlich gehalten:

1. Volle Anerkennung der BT als Futtermittel bereits im Broilermastbetrieb.
2. Verwendung von gutem gehäckselten Stroh.
3. Erreichung einer einheitlichen Struktur, Durchfeuchtung, positive Beeinflussung der im Tiefstreustapel ablaufenden enzymatischen Prozesse.
4. Ein möglichst weites Verhältnis von eingestreuter Strohmenge zu ausgestallter BT-Menge.
5. Sachgemäße Lagerung und Zwischenlagerung der BT nach der Ausstallung.

Es wird über Möglichkeiten eines breiteren Einsatzspektrums sowie über Erfahrungen bei der Silierung von BT mit Hackfrüchten und Mais berichtet. Hackfruchtmischsilagen mit BT sind positiv zu bewerten. Vornutzungsfärsen auf der Weide nahmen bei freiem Angebot und bei ausreichendem Weide-, Stroh- und Mineralstoffangebot BT-Mengen von 1–2,5 kg je Tier und Tag auf.
Schlußfolgerungen:
1. Futterwertprüfungen bei BT sind notwendig.
2. Wissenschaftliche Erkenntnisse über die Zusammenhänge zwischen Kot- und Strohanteil, Trockensubstanzgehalt und biologisch-enzymatische Einflüsse im BT-Stapel und Futterwert sind z. Zt. unzureichend.
3. Das Einsatzspektrum der BT sollte erweitert und die damit im Zusammenhang stehenden Fragen untersucht werden.

Agraringenieurschule „Theodor Roemer", Stadtroda[1]
Sektion Tierproduktion und Veterinärmedizin der Karl-Marx-Universität Leipzig, Wissenschaftsbereich Tierernährungschemie, Jena[2]

Elisabeth Flachowsky[1], R. Stubendorff[1], G. Cyriaci[2] und H.-J. Löhnert[2]

Neue Ergebnisse zum Einsatz von Broilertiefstreu in der Wiederkäuerfütterung

Da die in der DDR durchgeführten Versuche zur Nutzung von Broilertiefstreu (BT) als Futtermittel Ende der sechziger Jahre erfolgten, sollte durch neuere Untersuchungen ein Beitrag zur Einschätzung der veränderten Produktionsbedingungen in der Broilermast (z. B. Haltungsdauer, Rationsgestaltung, Besatzdichte, Einstreumaterial und -menge) auf Inhaltsstoffe und Futterwert der BT geleistet werden (Untersuchungszeitraum 1976–1983). Im Mittel enthielt die BT 786 g Trockensubstanz (TS) je kg Frischmasse; je kg TS waren 323 g Rohprotein, 14 g Rohfett, 165 g Rohfaser, 312 g N-freie Extraktstoffe und 177 g Rohasche enthalten. Folgender Mengen- und Spurenelementgehalt wurde ermittelt: Ca: 13; P: 11; Mg: 12; Na: 14; K: 20 g/kg TS; Fe: 1100; Mn: 250; Zn: 130; Cu: 105 mg/kg TS.

Sowohl die Angaben zu den erwähnten Inhaltsstoffen als auch die in 3 Versuchen an je 5 Hammeln ermittelte scheinbare Verdaulichkeit (organische Substanz: 71 %; Rohprotein: 66 %; Rohfett: 74 %; Rohfaser: 82 %; N-freie Extraktstoffe: 71 %) und die errechnete Energiekonzentation (454 EFr/kg TS) stimmen gut mit den Ergebnissen früherer Untersuchungen überein.

In sechs langfristigen Gruppenfütterungsversuchen (Tageszunahmen zwischen 608 und 1040 g/Tier) wurden unterschiedliche Anteile von BT in Mastrinderrationen geprüft sowie verschiedene Mineralstoff- und Vitamin-A-Ergänzungen vorgenommen. Bei Verfütterung einer Silage (100; 50 bzw. 0 %)-BT-Ration (0; 50 bzw. 100 % der TS aus Grobfutter) und geringen Konzentratgaben (2,0 kg/Tier und Tag) nahmen die Mastbullen 665; 735 bzw. 631 g/Tier und Tag zu.

Mit $\approx$0,5 kg BT je 100 kg Lebendmasse und Tag wird der Rohproteinbedarf von Mastrindern gedeckt. Zur Vermeidung von N- und P-Überschüssen ist der Anteil an BT in Mastrinderrationen zu begrenzen (<1 kg BT/100 kg Lebendmasse und Tag). BT kann auch in der Winterfütterung von Schafen eingesetzt werden.

Vor der Verfütterung sollte die BT mindestens zwei Wochen silageähnlich zwischengelagert werden.

Forschungszentrum für Tierproduktion Dummerstorf-Rostock der Akademie der Landwirtschaftswissenschaften der DDR, Bereich Tierernährung „Oskar Kellner“

A. Chudy

Computereinsatz in der Futterplanung

Die breite Einführung der dezentralisiert einsetzbaren Rechentechnik (Büro- und Personalcomputer) eröffnet der Tierernährungswissenschaft und insonderheit der Futterplanung neue Möglichkeiten für die Breitenanwendung ihrer Grundlagen, Kennzahlen und Methoden. Durch Übergabe periodisch aktualisierter Datenträger und Software können neue Erkenntnisse ohne Zeitverzug in die Praxis überführt werden, wobei der Umfang des Datenmaterials und der Kompliziertheitsgrad der Methoden gegenüber Vollständigkeit und Genauigkeit bzw. Spezifik und Praxisrelevanz ihrer Aussagen in den Hintergrund treten. Einmal von Spezialisten algorithmiert und programmiert ermöglicht die Anwendersoftware ihre tausendfache, von subjektiven Fehlern freie Anwendung.

Vorgestellt wurde ein kompatibeles Programmpaket, das die futterwirtschaftlichen Beziehungen von der Bodennutzung bis zur Rationsberechnung umfaßt und aus folgenden BC-Programmen bestehen wird:

1. Rationsberechnung und Futtereinsatzplanung ohne (RATBE I) und mit Angleichung der Rationen an einen vorgegebenen Futterfonds (RATBE II)
2. Planung und Bilanzierung von Futterbedarf und Futteraufkommen, getrennt nach Tierarten in bis zu 4 variabel vorgebbaren Zeitperioden (FPB1)
3. Futterverteilungs- und Futtereinsatzplanung mit zeitabhängiger und nach Tierkategorien getrennter Bilanzierung des Futtereinsatzes (FPB2)
4. Planung und Bilanzierung der Futterproduktion und des Futterflächenbedarfs (FUPRO)
5. Planung und Bilanzierung von Futterbedarf und Futterproduktion für Kooperationen (Territorien) mit zeitabhängiger Futterverteilung auf die Bedarfsträger (Tierkategorien) (FPB3 – als Kombination der Algorithmen von FPB2 und FUPRO).

Sektion Tierproduktion der Wilhelm-Pieck-Universität Rostock, Wissenschaftsbereich Tierernährung[1]
Tierkörperverarbeitungsbetrieb Malchin[2]

S. Poppe[1], Hanna Meier[1] und H. Kiehn[2]

Qualitätsgerechte Eiweißmischsilageproduktion und ihr Einsatz in der Fütterung

Mit der planmäßigen Steigerung der Tierproduktion in der DDR erhöht sich der Anfall von Abfallprodukten in der Schlachttierproduktion. In der Vergangenheit wurden aus den Abfallprodukten, wie Konfiskaten und Blut, in den Tierkörperverarbeitungsbetrieben (TKVB) Tierkörpermehl, Blutmehl und tierisches Rohfett hergestellt.

Mit steigender Tierproduktion mußte die Verarbeitungskapazität der TKVB erhöht werden. Dabei erwuchs die Aufgabe, ein Verfahren zu entwickeln, was einerseits die Verarbeitungskapazität erhöht, die Verluste an verdaulichem Rohprotein vermindert und außerdem die volkswirtschaftlich notwendige Tierfettproduktion ermöglicht. Durch das Verfahren der „Eiweißmischsilage" (EMS) wird diesen Forderungen zufriedenstellend und ökonomisch entsprochen. Bei der Herstellung der EMS wird das Absetzverfahren angewendet, da dadurch sehr unproblematisch das volkswirtschaftlich notwendige Tierkörperfett gewonnen werden kann. Außerdem ist das Absetzverfahren ökonomisch günstig, problemarm in der Anwendung und sichert bei richtiger Anwendung die angestrebten Futterwertparameter.

Hervorzuheben ist, daß mit der EMS-Produktion alle anfallenden tierischen Abfallprodukte, d. h. auch Blut, Fischabfälle und andere nicht traditionelle Rohstoffe, wie zum Beispiel Borsten, Fettschlamm, Chromleder, Federn, Darmschleim verarbeitet werden können.

Durch die neue Verarbeitungstechnologie erhöhte sich in der DDR von 1973 bis 1985 die Produktion an EMS von 5,1 kt auf 242,2 kt. Die Tierkörpermehlproduktion verringerte sich von 1973 bis 1985 von 34,8 kt auf 15,7 kt.

Der Futterwert der EMS hängt vor allem von ihrem Rohprotein- und Fettgehalt ab. Der Rohproteingehalt und seine Aminosäurenzusammensetzung ist im wesentlichen von den Komponenten abhängig, die zur Herstellung der EMS Verwendung finden.

Zur Charakterisierung des energetischen Futterwertes der EMS wurde die Verdaulichkeit der Hauptnährstoffe bestimmt. So beträgt die Verdaulichkeit der org. Subst. 75,2 %, des Rohproteins 83,5 % und die des Gesamtfetts 79,5 %.

Aus diesen Verdaulichkeitswerten wurde in Abhängigkeit vom Rohproteingehalt und vom Gehalt an Fett der energetische Futterwert berechnet. Daraus ist zu erkennen, daß bei ordnungsgemäßer Herstellung der EMS (10–12 % Rohprotein und 5–7 % Fett) mit einem Gehalt von 150–210 EF_s je kg gerechnet werden kann. Weiterhin ist auf Grund des günstigen Aminosäurenspektrums die Eiweißmischsilage geeignet, das Lysindefizit des Getreides in der Schweinefütterung nach kurzer Eingewöhnungszeit auszugleichen. Günstig ist es, mit der Silagefütterung schon im Läuferstadium zu beginnen und allmählich die Tiere an höhere Gaben zu gewöhnen. Eine diskontinuierliche Fütterung von EMS sollte generell vermieden werden, da sie in jedem Falle mit Leistungseinbußen verbunden ist.

Abschließend werden Angaben zur Einstufung der EMS in Qualitätsklassen entsprechend der TGL 38867 gemacht. Die Hauptursachen einer nicht TGL-gerechten EMS-Produktion liegen in Überschreitungen des Fettgehaltes (ca. 77 %) und Überschreitungen des pH-Wertes (27 %).

Sektion Tierproduktion und Veterinärmedizin der Karl-Marx-Universität Leipzig, Wissenschaftsbereich Tierfütterung und Ernährungsschäden[1]
VEB Fleischkombinat Leipzig[2]

M. Ulbrich[1] und P. Richter[2]

Erschließung und Nutzung von Futterreserven aus dem VEB Fleischkombinat Leipzig für die Kälberaufzucht

Mit der Inbetriebnahme einer Anlage zur Fettgewinnung im VEB SVB Leipzig, fallen Fette aus Rohstoffen an, die bisher nicht oder nur teilweise für Nahrungs- oder Futterzwecke zur Verfügung standen. Als Ausgangsmaterial dienen z. B. Croupon-, Schwarten- und Knochenfette sowie Fettabschnitte. Die Fettgemische entsprechen in ihrer Qualität den chemisch-physikalischen Daten, die als Anforderung an ein TGL-gerechtes Schweineschmalz gestellt werden. Unterschiedlich anfallendes Ausgangsmaterial führt zu Veränderungen im Fettsäuremuster, wobei besonders der Anteil an Ölsäure erhöht sein kann. In Versuchen sollte deshalb die Möglichkeit einer Nutzung dieser Fette zur Auffettung von Magermilch für die Kälberaufzucht geprüft werden. Dabei kamen Fette, wie Knochenfett und Rinderfußöl, zum Einsatz, um die Auswirkungen extrem hoher Ölsäuregehalte auf Verdauung und Wachstum der Kälber festzustellen. Für die Versuche wurden entsprechende Fettkonzentrate verwendet. Ein Verdauungsversuch mit 7 Wochen alten Kälbern ergab keine signifikanten Unterschiede in der Verdaulichkeit der organischen Substanz (92/93 %) einer Schmalz-Talg- gegenüber einer Knochenfettration, aber eine höhere Verdaulichkeit des Rohfettes in der Knochenfettgruppe (84/92 %). Im 60 Tage dauernden Wachstumsversuch mit den gleichen Fettkonzentraten traten keine signifikanten Unterschiede in den täglichen Lebendmassezunahmen (710 ± 70/674 ± 52 g) und im Energieaufwand (1,48 ± 0,11/1,51 ± 0,05 kEFr/kg LMZ) auf. In einem Gruppenfütterungsversuch mit Schmalz-Talg und den Extremvarianten Knochenfett bzw. Rinderfußöl betrugen die täglichen Lebendmassezunahmen in der 3. bis 11. Lebenswoche 582 ± 70/541 ± 58/541 ± 53 g und der Energieaufwand 1,65/1,76/1,76 kEFr/kg LMZ. Obwohl die Extremvarianten nicht für die Kälberaufzucht vorgesehen sind, zeigen die Versuche, daß die genannten Fette als Bestandteil von Fettgemischen ohne Nachteile verwendet werden können.

Sektion Tierproduktion und Veterinärmedizin der Karl-Marx-Universität Leipzig, Wissenschaftsbereich Tierernährungschemie, Jena

K. Gruhn und R. Zander

Neue Ergebnisse zur Verdaulichkeit der Rohnährstoffe und Aminosäuren von vorbehandelter und getrockneter Subkutis

Gegenwärtig werden in der DDR jährlich ≈ 3000 t geäscherte Subkutis bei der Lederherstellung anfallend, deponiert. Nach einem speziellen Aufbereitungsverfahren konnte ein trockenes Futtermittel folgender Zusammensetzung hergestellt werden (je kg Originalsubstanz): 939 g Trockensubstanz, 608 g Rohprotein, 96 g Rohfett, 43 g N-freie Extraktstoffe, 192 g Rohasche, 24,4 g Lysin, 11,2 g Methionin und 8,2 g Zystin. Die Daten stellen den Mittelwert aus 2 Chargen dar, deren scheinbare Verdaulichkeit der Rohnährstoffe an 22 kg schweren Börgen bzw. an kolostomierten Hennen und Hähnen der Legerichtung geprüft wurde. Die mittlere scheinbare Verdaulichkeit (in %) ist in der folgenden Tabelle aufgeführt:

	Schwein		Geflügel	
	$\bar{x}$	$s\pm$	$\bar{x}$	$s\pm$
Organische Substanz	79,2	6,8	77,1	0,6
Rohprotein	85,4	1,5	81,8	1,2
Rohfett	75,3	8,6	89,8	0,9
Lysin	84,9	1,7	84,4	1,2
Methionin	79,6	1,9	91,6	0,9
Zystin	84,8	1,1	60,8	1,6

Zwischen Hennen und Hähnen bestehen keine Unterschiede. Die scheinbare Verdaulichkeit der Rohnährstoffe und der erstlimitierenden Aminosäuren ist der der konventionellen Einweißfuttermittel gleichwertig. Aus den Ergebnissen wird geschlußfolgert, daß die aufbereitete Subkutis in der Tierfütterung eingesetzt werden kann. Für Mastschweine wird eine tägliche Gabe von 200–300 g/Tier empfohlen.

Sektion Tierproduktion und Veterinärmedizin der Karl-Marx-Universität Leipzig, Wissenschaftsbereich Tierernährungschemie, Jena

G. FLACHOWSKY und A. HENNIG

Futterwert von Fermentationsprodukten aus Tierexkrementen

Tierexkremente können durch aerobe und anaerobe Prozesse weiter aufbereitet und genutzt werden. Die Behandlung kann sowohl ohne als auch mit fremden C-Quellen erfolgen.

Die Fermentationsprodukte sind überwiegend N- und aschereicher als das verwendete Ausgangsmaterial, sie enthalten jedoch weniger fermentierbare Kohlenhydrate.

Der bei der aeroben Güllebehandlung (Oxidationsgraben, Oberflächenbelüftung) anfallende Belebtschlamm enthielt 40 bis 65 % Rohprotein und 20 bis 35 % Rohasche in der TS. In Hammelversuchen betrug die Verdaulichkeit der org. Subst. von Bioschlamm aus Schweinegülle 52 %, die des Rohproteins 70 %.

Legehennengülle-Stroh-Gemische wurden aerob fermentiert. Die Endprodukte enthielten 20 bis 25 % Rohprotein und >25 % Rohasche in der Trockensubstanz, die Verdaulichkeit der org. Sust. betrug beim Hammel 55 %.

Der Ablauf aus der Biogasproduktion ist proteinreich (25 bis 50 %), enthält jedoch auch 30 bis 40 % Rohasche in der TS. Für die Verdaulichkeit der org. Subst. wurden beim Wiederkäuer Werte zwischen 55 und 60 % ermittelt.

Die erwähnten Fermentationsprodukte haben gegenwärtig keine Bedeutung in der praktischen Fütterung.

Als weitere Fermentationsprodukte aus Tierexkrementen wurde der Futterwert von Algen, Fliegenpuppen und Regenwürmern eingeschätzt.

Algen (Chlorella, Scenedesmus u. a.) sind relativ proteinreich (35 bis 45 % Rohprotein in TS), die Abtrennung aus der Flüssigkeit bereitet jedoch erhebliche Schwierigkeiten. Der große Flächenbedarf, die erforderliche Temperatur und die relativ geringe Verdaulichkeit (54 bis 68 %) schränken ebenfalls die Bedeutung ein.

Fliegenpuppen und Regenwürmer sind proteinreich (60 bis 68 % der TS); der große Flächenbedarf, die geringe Exkrementumsetzung infolge der langsamen Entwicklung, die Ansprüche an die Temperatur und Schwierigkeiten bei der Sammlung begrenzen diese Methoden der Exkrementnutzung gegenwärtig auf Laborstudien.

Im Gegensatz zu Klärschlamm aus kommunalem Abwasser (mittlerer Gehalt: 5 mg Cd, 12 mg Hg, 150 mg Pb je kg TS) enthalten Fermentationsprodukte aus Tierexkrementen keine den Einsatz limitierende Schwermetallkonzentrationen.

Sektion Tierproduktion und Veterinärmedizin der Karl-Marx-Universität Leipzig, Wissenschaftsbereich Tierernährungsphysiologie und Futtermittelkunde

G. GEBHARDT und F. LIEBERT

Ergebnisse zur Wirksamkeit von Lysinkonzentrat als Lysinquelle für das wachsende Schwein

Für die Supplementation von zumeist Lysin limitierten Futtermittelmischungen für wachsende Schweine wird in der DDR der Einsatz eines mikrobiellen Lysinkonzentrates (ca. 30 g Lysin je 100 g Rohprotein) vorbereitet. Zur Quantifizierung der Lysinwirksamkeit wurden N-Umsatzmessungen an weiblichen Schweinen im Lebendmassebebereich von 30–45 kg durchgeführt. Dabei erfolgte auf Grundlage eines N-Verwertungsmodells der Vergleich mit der Wirksamkeit von nativem Lysin (Weizen, Weizenkleber) bzw. synthetischem Lysin (L-Lys · HCl). Folgende Hauptergebnisse sind aus den Untersuchungen ableitbar:

1. Bei 3maliger Futtergabe konnte für Lysinkonzentrat eine in der Tendenz geringfügig höhere Lysinwirksamkeit als für synthetisches Lysin festgestellt werden, lag aber nicht höher als im vergleichend geprüften Weizenkleberprotein.
2. Eine Differenzierung der Fütterungshäufigkeit (2 bzw. 5) ergab bei 5maliger Fütterung in der Tendenz einen positiven Effekt auf die Lysinwirksamkeit von synthetischem Lysin, nicht aber beim Lysinkonzentrat.
3. Die Untersuchung von Lysinkonzentrat lieferte einen mittleren Lysinwirkungskoeffizienten für die geprüften Produkte (ČSSR bzw. DDR-Produktion) von $k = 0{,}87$, der ein hohes Niveau der Lysinwirksamkeit ausweist, zugleich aber auch unterstreicht, daß nicht von einer 100 %igen Lysinbereitstellung aus Lysinkonzentrat ausgegangen werden kann.

Insgesamt zeigen die Ergebnisse aus ernährungsphysiologischer Sicht, daß Lysinkonzentrat mikrobieller Herkunft eine gute Lysinquelle für das Schwein darstellt und daß bei homogener Einbringung in entspr. Futtermischungen keine zusätzlichen Anforderungen an die Häufigkeit der Fütterung vorliegen. Analoge Schlußfolgerungen konnten aus der Supplementation von Corn-Cob-Mix(CCM)-Silage mit Lysinkonzentrat bzw. synthetischem Lysin beim Schwein abgeleitet werden.

Forschungszentrum für Tierproduktion Dummerstorf-Rostock der Akademie der Landwirtschaftswissenschaften der DDR, Bereich Tierernährung „Oskar Kellner"

L. SCHMIDT, F. WEISSBACH und B. REUTER

Weiterentwicklung der Welksilageproduktion durch Anwendung von Siliermitteln

Durch den Einsatz von Siliermitteln soll das Welkverfahren, das nach wie vor das wichtigste Silierverfahren ist, nicht abgelöst, sondern dahingehend verbessert werden, daß bei ungünstigen Welkbedingungen auch unterhalb des sonst erforderlichen Mindest-Trockensubstanzgehaltes mit Erfolg siliert werden kann. Der erforderliche Mindest-Trockensubstanzgehalt ist von der Vergärbarkeit des Grünfutters (gekennzeichnet durch den Z/PK-Quotienten) abhängig. Die in umfangreichen Laborversuchen nachgewiesene Wirkung der aus einheimischen Rohstoffen herstellbaren flüssigen Siliermittel Cekafusil und Natriumpyrosulfitlösung ist der Wirkung einer Erhöhung des Trockensubstanzgehaltes um etwa 10 % (absolut) äquivalent. Die Konzeption des Siliermitteleinsatzes sieht deshalb die Kombination mit schwachem Welken auf 20–30 % TS-Gehalt (anstelle von 30–40 % TS bisher) vor. Damit können die Feldliegezeit auf 1–2 Tage verkürzt und die Feldverluste vermindert werden.

Für die Applikation der Siliermittel ist in Zusammenarbeit mit dem FZM Schlieben/Bornim eine Technologie entwickelt worden, die die Dosierung am Feldhäcksler ermöglicht. Der Einsatz o. gen. Siliermittel nach dieser Technologie hat sich in Produktionsexperimenten gut bewährt. Bei der Silierung von etwa 44000 t Grünfutter wurden zu 95 % sehr gute und gute Silagen erhalten.

Sektion Tierproduktion der Wilhelm-Pieck-Universität Rostock, Wissenschaftsbereich Tierernährung

W. Wiesemüller

Ergebnisse und Erfahrungen bei der Silierung eiweißreicher Futterpflanzen

Seit 1984 werden Versuche zur Applikation heißer verdünnter H_2SO_4 auf den Feldbestand von Futterpflanzen zum Zweck ihrer Silierung durchgeführt. Dafür wird ein Gerätesystem zur Abtötung von Kartoffelkraut genutzt, das mit Keramikdüsen bestückt wird, welche eine Dosierung von 3 Liter H_2SO_4/t Grünmasse ermöglichen. Das sind 11 mVal/100 kg Grünfutter bzw. 60 % der Säuremenge des Verfahrens von A. I. Virtanen. Nach der Säureapplikation tritt ein Sikkationseffekt auf. Der TS-Gehalt der Pflanzen erhöht sich in 16 h um absolut 5 %. Etwa 4 h nach der Säurebehandlung ist die Schwefelsäure von der Blattoberfläche aufgenommen. Während Sikkation und Nachwelken geht keine Säure verloren; der osmotische Druck steigt im Pflanzensaft. Versuche mit Luzerne, Klee, Knaulgras, Lupinen, Futterroggen und Wiesengras ergaben Silagen, die weniger als 4 g Buttersäure/kg TS und unter 5 % NH_3-N im Kjeldahl-N enthielten, wobei der Reinproteinverlust gegenüber dem grünen Ausgangsmaterial im Durchschnitt bei nur 15 % lag. Die applizierte Schwefelsäure schädigte in keinem Fall den Nachwuchs mehrschnittiger und mehrjähriger Futterpflanzen. Vermehrungsrotklee, dessen 1. Schnitt nach diesem Verfahren behandelt wurde, ergab außergewöhnlich gute Saatguterträge. Das Verfahren ermöglicht eine Vorverlegung des ersten Schnittes sowie eine sichere Konservierung der Zwischenfrüchte und des 4. Schnittes im Oktober. Von den 1985 wissenschaftlich betreuten 25000 t Versuchssilagen hatten über 95 % die Siliernote 1.

In Fütterungsversuchen erhielten Milchkühe 5 kg Silage-TS/Tag in Verbindung mit einer zweiten Silage über einen längeren Zeitraum mit einer positiven Auswirkung auf die Milchqualität. An 1600 Jungrinder einer Anlage wurde 50 % der verzehrten Futter-Trockensubstanz Kleegras-Schwefelsäuresilage über 100 Tage eingesetzt. Am Ende des Versuches wurden im Harn pH = 8,1 und NSBA + 123 mmol/L sowie im Serum ein Kupfergehalt von 15,9 µmol/L ermittelt, was darauf hinweist, daß der

Sulfatschwefelgehalt von 6–10/kg TS in der Silage bei richtiger Dosierung eines Mineralstoffgemisches problemlos ist. An 150 Sauen wurden ganzjährig über 15 Monate 4 kg Luzernesilage/Tag eingesetzt, wobei gute Fruchtbarkeitsleistungen und Stoffwechselparameter erzielt wurden.

Im Rahmen des staatlichen Zulassungsverfahrens werden 1986/87 in Zusammenarbeit mit der Chemieberatungsstelle Halle und Einrichtungen des Veterinärwesens und des Umweltschutzes die Prüfungen fortgesetzt.

Forschungszentrum für Tierproduktion Dummerstorf-Rostock der Akademie der Landwirtschaftswissenschaften der DDR, Bereich Tierernährung „Oskar Kellner"

B. Piatkowski und J. Voigt

Zur Bedeutung der Mineralsäure-Silage aus eiweißreichem Grünfutter

Der relativ hohe Anteil an buttersäurehaltigen Silagen aus eiweißreichem Grünfutter verschlechtert die Energieeinnahme, die Rohproteinversorgung, die Rohmilchqualität und die Gesundheit der Kühe besonders im geburtsnahen Zeitraum. Neben der bisher üblichen Herstellung von Welksilage (35–45 % TS) wird die Anwendung der chemischen Konservierung notwendig. Das neu entwickelte Siliermittel „Cekafusil" hat seine größte Wirksamkeit im TS-Bereich von 25–35 %. Da für das Siliergut mit 15–20 % sowie bei auftretendem Regen infolge des Fehlens von Ameisensäure kein alternatives Siliermittel vorhanden ist, wurden ab 1980 Mineralsäuren entsprechend der AIV-Methode sowie in verschiedenen Gemischen geprüft.
In einem Experiment an 4 Kühen mit Duodenalbrückenfistel und einer Leistung von 24 kg Milch (4 % Fett) wurde die Ration mit Graswelksilage (37 % TS) und 2,5 kg Sojaextraktionsschrot durch eiweißreiche Kleesilage (20 % TS) konserviert mit $H_2SO_4 + HCOOH$ ausgetauscht. Dabei wurden folgende Ergebnisse erhalten:

	Welksilage	Kleesilage
TS-Aufnahme, kg	16,6 ± 1,68	16,7 ± 0,93
N-Aufnahme, g	445 ± 58	430 ± 25
NAN am Duodenum, g	449 ± 73	451 ± 34
g je kg TS-Aufnahme am Duodenum	27,1	27,0

Von der mit H_2SO_4 + Ameisensäure konservierten Kleesilage mit 19,6 % Rohprotein wurden 7,6 kg TS täglich aufgenommen, wodurch eine vergleichbare duodenale Rohproteinversorgung auch ohne Extraktionsschrot vorlag.

Am Beispiel der landwirtschaftlichen Kooperation Lüssow Krs. Güstrow (2100 Kühe 6000 t Mineralsäure (MS) Silage pro Jahr) konnte nach zweijähriger Fütterung (3–4 kg TS MS-Silage je Tag und Kuh) ein deutlicher Leistungsanstieg je Tier, eine verbesserte Stoffwechsellage der Herde sowie eine bedeutsame Verbesserung der Rohmilchqualität (Klasse Qu von 80 auf 99 %) erreicht werden. Die angewandte Technologie (Besprühen des Siliergutes vor dem Silo mit Hilfe des Häckselers E 280 wurde weiter verbessert und erlaubt die tägliche Silierung von 500 t. Die notwendigen Vorschriften für den Bau und Betrieb der Säuremischstationen liegen in Form einer Verfahrensbeschreibung mit bestätigter Schutzgüte vor. Zur Produktion von buttersäurefreien Silagen wird es zukünftig notwendig sein, unter unseren Bedingungen der Futterproduktion und Materialbereitstellung in Ergänzung der Welksilierung die verschiedensten Möglichkeiten der chemischen Konservierung je nach Futterart, Standort und Witterung zu nutzen.

Posterdiskussion

Forschungszentrum für Tierproduktion Dummerstorf-Rostock der Akademie der Landwirtschaftswissenschaften der DDR, Bereich Tierernährung „Oskar Kellner“

H.-J. Block und F. Weissbach

Chemische Veränderungen der Zellwandsubstanzen beim Strohaufschluß mit NH_3 aus Harnstoff

Die Veränderungen der Zellwandsubstanzen beim Strohaufschluß mit NH_3 aus Harnstoff sind von der Aufschlußtemperatur abhängig.

Bei Erwärmung ≤ 15 °C ändern sich Gehalt und Wasserlöslichkeit der Zellwandsubstanzen (Lignin, Rohzellulosen, Hemizellulosen) nicht. Eine Steigerung der Lagerungstemperatur bis 75 °C führt zu einem kontinuierlichen Anstieg im Ligningehalt (Artefaktligninbildung) und zu einer deutlichen Abnahme im Hemizellulosengehalt (thermische Kondensation zu Artefaktlignin und Reaktion der Pentosen mit NH_3). Demgegenüber ist der Zuwachs im Rohzellulosegehalt relativ gering.

Über 25 °C werden die Hemizellulosen leicht unter Freisetzung von Azetat entazetyliert. Mit zunehmender Aufschlußtemperatur werden solche Prozesse intensiviert, die zur Zerstörung der Zellwände führen. Das äußert sich in einem linearen Anstieg der Wasserlöslichkeit der org. Subst., die auf der Freisetzung eines löslichen Lignin-Hemizellulosen-Komlexes bzw. löslicher Lignin- und Hemizellulosenbausteine beruht. Mit zunehmender Aufschlußintensität steigt das Ausmaß der Stickstoffbindung aus dem NPN-Zusatz deutlich an. Der Hauptteil dieses N liegt bei milden Bedingungen (≤ 25 °C) als wasserlösliches Ammonium, bei Erhitzung über 50 °C jedoch in wachsendem Maße in der Ligninfraktion gebunden vor.

Forschungszentrum für Tierproduktion Dummerstorf-Rostock der Akademie der Landwirtschaftswissenschaften der DDR, Bereich Tierernährung „Oskar Kellner“

E. Bergner, F. Weissbach und H. Cöster

Futteraufnahme, Mastleistung und Energieaufwand beim Einsatz von harnstoffbehandeltem Stroh im Rindermastversuch

Je 9 SMR-Jungbullen ($\bar{x}$ 175 kg Anfangslebendmasse) erhielten zu einer Ration von 1,5 kg Gerstenschrot und 9 kg Zuckerrübenblattsilage als Versuchsgruppe harnstoffbehandeltes und als Kontrollgruppe unbehandeltes, gehäckseltes Winterroggenstroh. Alle Tiere wurden mit 440 kg Lebendmasse geschlachtet und einer Ganzkörperanalyse unterzogen.

Als Versuchsfutter wurde erntefrisches, trockenes Roggenstroh auf 35–40 % aufgefeuchtet, mit 3 % Harnstoff vermischt und im Horizontalsilo eingelagert. Die Energiekonzentration betrug 432 EFr/kg TS bei der Verfütterung. Kontrollfutter war Stroh vom gleichen Ernteschlag, geborgen nach Einregnen im Schwad und Wiederabtrocknen. Die EK betrug 288 EFr/kg TS.

Ergebnisse ($\bar{x}$ $n = 9$ je Gruppe): Der Aufschlußeffekt im Harnstoffstroh und die um 0,63 kg TS/Tier/d höhere Strohaufnahme der Versuchstiere führten zur Erhöhung der Masttagszunahmen um 123 g, zur Verkürzung der Mastdauer um 47 Tage und zur Senkung des Konzentrataufwandes um 17 % gegenüber der Kontrollgruppe. Der TS-Aufwand je kg Lebendmassezunahme war bei den Versuchstieren um 0,89 kg geringer, der Energieaufwand um 0,37 kEFr höher. Je Masttag wurden 11 g Protein, 50 g Fett und 2,29 MJ Energie mehr angesetzt als bei den Kontrolltieren. Alle Unterschiede waren signifikant ($\alpha = 0{,}05$).

Forschungszentrum für Tierproduktion Dummerstorf-Rostock der Akademie der Landwirtschaftswissenschaften der DDR, Bereich Tierernährung „Oskar Kellner“ [1]
Forschungszentrum für Mechanisierung der Landwirtschaft Schlieben/Bornim, Abteilung Abtshagen [2]

L. SCHMIDT [1], F. WEISSBACH [1] und H. STROMEYER [2]

Konservierung und chemischer Aufschluß von Stroh in Quadergroßballen durch Harnstoffzusatz

Die Herstellung von hochverdichteten Quadergroßballen aus Stroh ist ein technologisch und ökonomisch vorteilhaftes Verfahren der Strohbergung und Strohlagerung, das künftig auch in der DDR angewendet werden soll. Ein entsprechendes Verfahren wurde vom Forschungszentrum für Mechanisierung der Landwirtschaft Schlieben-Bornim entwickelt. Allerdings sind die Anforderungen für eine qualitätsgerechte und verlustarme Lagerung der Großballen in bezug auf den zulässigen Wassergehalt des Strohs höher als bei herkömmlichen Strohbergungsverfahren, wenn das Großballenstroh nicht chemisch konserviert wird. Durch die Verwendung von Harnstoff als Konservierungsmittel ist es gelungen, Quadergroßballen mit Strohfeuchten bis zu 50 % lagerfähig zu machen. Der Konservierungseffekt beruht auf der Freisetzung von Ammoniak bei der Harnstoffhydrolyse, die in feuchten Futtermitteln spontan erfolgt. Ammoniak ist eine stark fungizide Substanz, die insbesondere Schimmelpilze abtötet, aber auch die Entwicklung von Bakterien hemmt. Gleichzeitig ist Ammoniak aber auch ein Aufschlußmittel zur Erhöhung der Verdaulichkeit des Strohs und eine NPN-Quelle für die Pansenproteinsynthese.

Zur Gewährleistung des Konservierungserfolges werden im Feuchtebereich zwischen 15 und 50 % je 1 % Strohfeuchte 0,1 % Harnstoff benötigt. Damit wurde bei Strohfeuchten von durchschnittlich 30 % ein mittlerer Aufschlußeffekt von 60 EFr/kg TS erzielt. Fast 40 % des zugesetzten NPN blieben in den konservierten Quadergroßballen als NPN-Quelle für die Pansenproteinsynthese erhalten.

Forschungszentrum für Tierproduktion Dummerstorf-Rostock der Akdademie der Landwirtschaftswissenschaften der DDR, Bereich Tierernährung „Oskar Kellner“ [1]
Institut für Futterproduktion Paulinenaue der Akademie der Landwirtschaftswissenschaften der DDR [2]

L. SCHMIDT [1], F. WEISSBACH [1], H. LETTOW [2] und H. THÖNS [2]

Konservierung und chemischer Aufschluß von Stroh bei silageähnlicher Lagerung durch Harnstoffzusatz

Mit Harnstoff behandeltes feuchtes Futterstroh im Feuchtebereich zwischen 30 und 60 % wird in ähnlicher Weise wie Siliergut aus Grünfutter in Horizontal- und Hochslios eingelagert, verdichtet und zugedeckt. Dieses Verfahren, das mit vorhandener Technik durchgeführt werden kann, hat sich bereits in vielen Produktionsbetrieben bewährt.

Harnstoffzusätze zum feuchten Stroh verhindern den aeroben und anaeroben Verderb, schließen das Stroh auf und reichern es mit NPN an.

Die erforderliche Harnstoffdosis (bezogen auf feuchtes Stroh) beträgt 3 % bei Strohfeuchten bis 50 % und 4 % bei Strohfeuchten über 50 %.

Unbehandeltes feuchtes Stroh neigt bei anaerober Lagerung und Strohfeuchten über 40 % zur Buttersäuregärung. Modellversuche haben gezeigt, daß die Buttersäurebildung durch Harnstoffzusatz gehemmt werden kann. Gegen Schimmelbildung ist harnstoffbehandeltes Stroh auch in Silos bei Luftzutritt bzw. nach der Auslagerung zuverlässig geschützt.

Die Verdaulichkeit und damit die Energiekonzentration des harnstoffbehandelten Strohs war durchschnittlich um 1/3 höher als die des unbehandelten Ausgangsmaterials (um etwa 100 EFr/kg TS).

Vom zugesetzten Harnstoffstickstoff wurden durchschnittlich 69 % im Konservat wiedergefunden. Davon waren 25 % unverdaulich, so daß 44 % als NPN für die Pansenproteinsynthese erhalten blieben.

Forschungszentrum für Tierproduktion Dummerstorf-Rostock der Akademie der Landwirtschaftswissenschaften der DDR, Bereich Tierernährung „Oskar Kellner“

H.-J. Block und F. Weissbach

Einfluß von Harnstoff bei der silageähnlichen Lagerung von Feuchtstroh auf die Gärsäurenbildung

Im Rahmen der Untersuchungen zur Konservierung von feuchtem Futterstroh mit Harnstoff wurde festgestellt, daß ein Harnstoffzusatz durch das sehr schnell auf ureolytischem Wege freigesetzte Ammoniak die mikrobielle Gärung hemmt und zu alkalischen Konservaten führt (pH > 8). Der Hauptteil an Essigsäure in harnstoffkonserviertem Stroh entsteht auf chemischem Wege durch Azetylgruppenabspaltung aus den Hemizellulosen.

Sowohl Milchsäurebildung als auch n-Buttersäuregärung werden bei ausreichender Harnstoffdosierung unterbunden. Der Konservierungseffekt von Harnstoffzusätzen ist entscheidend vom Wassergehalt des zu konservierenden Strohes abhängig. In Modellversuchen reichten bei >60 % Feuchte 2,5 % Harnstoff (auf Orig.substanz Stroh), von 40 ... 60 % Feuchte 2,0 % Harnstoff zur Unterdrückung einer Buttersäurebildung. Strohfeuchten <30 % erforderten hierzu keinen Harnstoffzusatz. Unter praktischen Silierbedingungen sind jedoch Sicherheitszuschläge hinsichtlich der Höhe des Harnstoffzusatzes notwendig.

Sektion Tierproduktion und Veterinärmedizin der Karl-Marx-Universität Leipzig, Wissenschaftsbereich Tierernährungschemie, Jena [1]
Rowett Research Institute, Aberdeen [2]

G. Flachowsky [1] und E. R. Ørskov [2]

Nylonbeutel-Trockensubstanzverlust von Milchkuhkot, der nach Fütterung von unbehandeltem bzw. NH_3-begastem Winter- bzw. Sommergerstenstroh anfiel

Frischkot sowie der wasserunlösliche Rückstand von Milchkuhkot wurde in Nylonbeutel gegeben und 8; 16; 24; 48; 72 bzw. 96 h in den Pansen von drei Schafen inkubiert. Der Kot stammte von Kühen, die eine lose Schüttmischung, bestehend aus 50 % Konzentrat und 50 % unterschiedlich behandeltem Stroh, ad libitum verzehren konnten.

Als Stroh kam unbehandeltes Wintergerstenstroh (1), mit 3 % NH_3 behandeltes Wintergerstenstroh (2), unbehandeltes Sommergerstenstroh (3) bzw. mit 3 % NH_3 behandeltes Sommergerstenstroh (4) zum Einsatz.

Nach 48 h Pansen-Inkubationszeit betrug der Trockensubstanzverlust des Kotes (1 bis 4) 49,2; 58,5; 59,9 bzw. 64,7 %, vom wasserunlöslichen Rückstand waren 18,3; 30,9; 23,6 bzw. 29,5 % verschwunden. Nach 96 h Inkubationszeit betrug der Trockensubstanzverlust des wasserunlöslichen Rückstandes 30,2; 44,2; 35,5 bzw. 46,4 % (1 bis 4). Demnach ist Kot von Milchkühen, die NH_3-behandeltes Stroh verzehrten, eine effektivere Energiequelle für Rezyklierung und Methanproduktion bzw. ein besseres Nährsubstrat für Pilze im Vergleich zu unbehandeltem Stroh. Kot, der nach Fütterung von Sommergerstenstroh anfiel, besitzt im Vergleich zu Wintergerstenstroh ein höheres Fermentationspotential.

Sektion Tierproduktion und Veterinärmedizin der Karl-Marx-Universität Leipzig, Wissenschaftsbereich Tierernährungschemie, Jena

R. Schubert, J. Schwartze und R. Fuchs

Untersuchungen zum Futterwert von NH_3-begastem Stroh für Pferde

Jeweils vier Haflinger-Wallache und eine Stute erhielten über einen Zeitraum von 80 Tagen eine konstante Mischfuttergabe (Hafer 940, Sojaextraktionsschrot 40, Mineralstoffgemisch 10, Mileipan 10 g/kg) von 3,4 kg/100 kg $LM^{0,75}$/d und entweder mit 3 % NH_3 begastem oder unbehandeltes scheunengelagertes Weizenhäckselstroh ad libitum. Die Verdaulichkeit der gemischten Rationen mit jeweils 15 % Stroh wurde an je 3 Ponys ermittelt. Im Mittel des Versuches verzehrten die Haflinger je Tier täglich 5 kg TS aus NH_3-Stroh bzw. 4,5 kg TS aus unbehandeltem Stroh (54 bzw. 49 g TS/kg $LM^{0,75}$).

Die Tiere der Gruppe, die NH_3-begastes Stroh erhielten, nahmen im Mittel des Versuches 93 g/Tier und Tag weniger an Lebendmasse ab als die Kontrolltiere. Die Verdaulichkeit der organischen Substanz gemischter Rationen mit 15 % NH_3-begastem Stroh für Ponys war um 12 % (relativ) höher als bei gleichem Anteil an unbehandeltem Stroh.

Staatliches Institut für Epizootiologie und Tierseuchenbekämpfung, Wusterhausen[1]
Sektion Tierproduktion und Veterinärmedizin der Humboldt-Universität zu Berlin, Wissenschaftsbereich Tierfütterung und Ernährungsschäden[2]

J. Teuffert[1], L. Hasselmann[2] und B. Raue[1]

Vergleichende Untersuchungen zum Einsatz von traditionellem Trockengrobfutter und verschieden behandelten Strohmaterialien in der Kälberfütterung

Mit den Untersuchungen verband sich die Zielstellung, die hinsichtlich Futteraufnahme, Lebendmasseentwicklung, Konzentrateinsparung und Durchfallprophylaxe in der Ferkel- und Läuferaufzucht erfolgreich eingesetzten Strohmaterialien auf ihre Eignung als Alternative zur Heufütterung in der Kälberaufzucht zu prüfen. Dazu wurden 34 männl. Kälber der Genotypen 30–35 mit einem mittleren Lebensalter von 14 Tagen in Einzelhaltung aufgestallt und in 4 Fütterungsgruppen eingeteilt. Alle Kälber erhielten im K1-Bereich Kälmil-Wassertränke (1:10) und Kälberaufzuchtfutter (pelletiert) lt. TGL 22256/01 und zusätzlich Grobfutter ad libitum. Im K2-Bereich entfiel die Kälmil-Wassertränke. Das Grobfutter bestand in der FG I (Fütterungsgruppe) aus Heumehl, in der FG II aus Strohmehl unbehandelt, in der FG III aus HCl-behandeltem Strohmehl und in der FG IV aus teilhydrolysiertem Strohmehl (Siebgröße 10 mm, Hammermühle). Die Versuchsdauer betrug 77 Haltungstage; ab 99. Lebenstag Vorperiode und Bilanzversuch. In 4wöchentlichem Abstand wurden jeweils 22 Blutparameter, 9 Harnparameter, 9 Kotparameter und die Pansenfermentation untersucht. Sowohl die Grobfutteraufnahme als auch die Lebendmasseentwicklung in den Fütterungsgruppen HCl-Strohmehl sowie teilhydrolysiertes Strohmehl ist unbefriedigend und der Heumehl- und unbeh. Strohmehlgruppe signifikant unterlegen. Der Einsatz von unbehandeltem Strohmehl zeigt zufriedenstellende Ergebnisse.

Sektion Tierproduktion und Veterinärmedizin der Humboldt-Universität zu Berlin, Bereich Tierernährung

R. SCHWEITZER und A. PÜSCHNER

Beeinflussung der Verschwindensrate von VOT bei unterschiedlicher Behandlung von Rapsextraktionsschrot-Strohmehl-Gemischen

In in-vitro-Untersuchungen wurde die Wirkung einer unterschiedlichen Behandlung von Rapsextraktionsschrot-Strohmehl-Gemischen auf die Verschwindensrate von 5-Vinyl-oxazolidin-2-thion (VOT) geprüft.

Unter Variation der Faktoren Mischungsverhältnis (RES : Strohmehl), Säurekonzentration (HCl), Einwirkzeit der Säure in einem geschlossenen System bei Raumtemperatur, Dämpfzeit unter Säurewirkung in einem geschlossenen System bei T = 105 °C und Lagerzeit des behandelten Gemisches in einem offenen System bei Raumtemperatur wurde der Einfluß der einzelnen Parameter auf die Änderung des Gehaltes an VOT ermittelt.

Bei Erhöhung der Behandlungsparameter konnte in allen Fällen ein Anstieg der Verschwindensrate verzeichnet werden. Die Veränderung von Säurekonzentration, Lagerzeit und Dämpfzeit beeinflußte den Anstieg der Verschwindensrate stärker als die Variation von Einwirkzeit und Mischungsverhältnis. Bei Minimierung eines Einflußfaktors verminderte sich die Wirkung der anderen Parameter auf die Änderung der Verschwindensrate.

Sektion Tierproduktion und Veterinärmedizin der Karl-Marx-Universität Leipzig, Wissenschaftsbereich Tierernährungschemie, Jena [1]
Rowett Research Institute, Aberdeen [2]

G. FLACHOWSKY [1], E. R. ØRSKOV [2]

Trockensubstanzverlust von Gerstenstroh im Pansen vor und nach Ernte des Speisepilzes Pleurotus ostreatus

Gerstenstroh wurde angefeuchtet (≈40 % TS), mit Sporen des eßbaren Pilzes Pleurotus ostreatus versetzt und in verschlossenen Plastesäcken bei Zimmertemperatur drei Monate gelagert. Nach Entwicklung des Myzels wurde die Plaste entfernt, so daß die Pilze wachsen konnten. Nach Pilzernte wurden der Rückstand sowie Ausgangsstroh und Stroh nach Myzelwachstum schonend getrocknet, gemahlen und zur Bestimmung des Trockensubstanzverlustes im Schafpansen mit Hilfe der Nylonbeutel-Methode aufbereitet (Einwaage: 2 g je Beutel). Die Pansen-Inkubationszeiten betrugen 8; 16; 24; 48; 72 bzw. 96 h. Die Schafe wurden mit gehäckseltem Heu gefüttert (1,3 kg/Tier und Tag).

Die Wasserlöslichkeit, die nach Waschen von Strohproben in Nylonbeuteln ermittelt wurde, war für Stroh nach Myzelwachstum bzw. nach Pilzernte (13,9 bzw. 15,2 %) signifikant höher als von Ausgangsstroh (8,9 %). Nach 8 Stunden Panseninkubationszeit bestanden keine wesentlichen Unterschiede im Trockensubstanzverlust, nach 48 h war der Abbau beim Ausgangsstroh (48,0 %) signifikant höher als nach Myzelwachstum bzw. Pilzernte (35,1 bzw. 30,4 %).

Nach diesen Ergebnissen sollten die Strohrückstände nach Pleurotus-Wachstum vorrangig als Dünger genutzt werden.

Sektion Tierproduktion und Veterinärmedizin der Karl-Marx-Universität Leipzig, Wissenschaftsbereich Tierernährungsphysiologie und Futtermittelkunde[1] sowie Tierernährungschemie[2]
LPG „Aufbau" Steutz, Geflügelversuchsanlage Jütrichau[3]

M. ABOUD[1], H. JEROCH[1], K. GRUHN[2] und K.-H. ENGERER[3]

Futterwert von CCM-Silage für das Geflügel und Einsatzprüfung von CCM-Rationen in der Broilermast

In Versuchen mit kolostomierten Hennen wurde die Verdaulichkeit von CCM-Silage mit 70 g (hoher Spindelanteil) bzw. 41 g Rohfaser (niedriger Spindelanteil) ermittelt, deren Ausgangsmaterial über 6- bzw. 10-mm-Siebe (Partikelanteil 2 mm 71–76 % bzw. 24–29 %) zerkleinert wurde. Die Verdaulichkeit der OS beträgt 78 % (70 g RFa) bzw. 85 % (41 g RFa). Auf der Grundlage der experimentellen Verdauungswerte errechnet sich eine Energiekonzentration (EFh/kg TS) von 718 (70 g RFa) bzw. 789 (41 g RFa). Der unterschiedliche Zerkleinerungsgrad hatte keinen Einfluß auf den Futterwert der geprüften CCM-Silagen.

Die Substitution von Körnermais durch CCM-Silage mit hohem bzw. niedrigem Rohfasergehalt in konventionellen Broilermastmischungen (Proteinträger: Sojaex.schrot, Fischmehl, Futterhefe) ergab im Mittel von 2 Versuchen mit männlichen Tieren 42tägiger Mastdauer folgendes Resultat: 1884 g (Maisgruppe), 1748 g (CCM mit 70 g RFa) bzw. 1855 g Mastendmasse (41 g RFa). Der Aufwand an Futtertrockensubstanz je kg Zunahme betrug in gleicher Gruppenfolge 2,04, 2,18 bzw. 1,95 kg.

Wissenschaftlich Technisches Zentrum des VEB Broiler- und Gänseproduktion Mockrehna

H. BERGER

Einsatz von CCM-Silage bei Legegänsen (Erste Ergebnisse)

Die Untersuchungen hatten das Ziel, CCM-Silage als Komponente zur günstigeren Gestaltung des Eiweiß-Energie-Verhältnisses in der Ration für Legegänse (ČSSR-Genotyp 003) bzw. als zusätzlichen Linolsäureträger zu prüfen.

CCM-Silage (10 mm – Teilchengröße) wurde zusätzlich ad libitum zum Mischfutter (ZG) gereicht (II), bzw. im Gemisch mit einem Eiweißkonzentrat, ergänzt durch Mineralstoff- und Wirkstoffmischung, angeboten (III). Die ersten Ergebnisse (im Kurztest von 9 Legewochen) weisen darauf hin, daß mit beiden Prüfvarianten, verglichen mit einer Kontrollgruppe (I), die ZG ad libitum erhielt, eine höhere Legeleistung (+4 bis +8 %), eine Verbesserung der Befruchtung und damit ein höherer Anteil an Gösseln je Gans erzielt werden können.

Der Rohproteinverzehr war um 3 bis 12 % verringert. Mit Variante II konnte zudem eine Einsparung an Mischfutter (ZG) bis 15 % erreicht werden.

Sektion Tierproduktion und Veterinärmedizin der Karl-Marx-Universität Leipzig, Wissenschaftsbereich Tierernährungsphysiologie und Futtermittelkunde

F. REINISCH, DIANA BERNDT, C. WECKE und G. GEBHARDT

Einsatz von CCM bei Ferkeln

Der Futterwert von 3 CCM-Varianten (normaler Hybridmais, derselbe einschließlich 10 % Luzerneblätter, lysinreiche Maismutante) wurde im einfachen Verdauungsversuch an Ferkeln (7 bis 10 kg LM) bestimmt sowie vergleichsweise an Mastschweinen mit etwa 95 kg LM. Die Energiekonzentration beträgt 738 (Mastschwein 742), 718 (741) bzw. 719 (725). Ferkel verdauen insbesondere das Rohprotein der CCM-Silage um 11 bis 16 Prozentpunkte geringer, wodurch die Proteinkonzentration nur 70, 69 bzw. 58 erreicht gegenüber 81, 86 bzw. 74 beim Mastschwein. Im Wachstumsversuch von der 6. bis einschließlich 10. Lebenswoche mit diesen CCM-Varianten und „Vormischung für CCM-Fütterung an Ferkel" (Mischungsverhältnis 1 : 1, jeweils äquivalente Lysinversorgung) erzielte Tageszunahmen von 458, 474 bzw. 433 g entsprechen der FA-I-Kontrolle mit 457 g. Mit 1,18; 1,13 bzw. 1,24 kEFs Energieaufwand gegenüber 1,30 der Kontrolle erreichen mit CCM gefütterte Ferkel einen signifikant verringerten Energieaufwand, vor allem durch Stabilisierung der Verdauung bzw. Kotkonsistenz, sicherlich in Verbindung mit dem Milchsäuregehalt von 15 bis 20 g/kg CCM.

Sektion Tierproduktion und Veterinärmedizin der Karl-Marx-Universität Leipzig, Wissenschaftsbereich Tierernährungsphysiologie und Futtermittelkunde

F. LIEBERT, R. KOHL und G. GEBHARDT

Futterwert von teilentschälter Gerste beim Ferkel

Vergleichend wurden Gerste, teilentschälte Gerste und Weizen als Einzelfuttermittel im Verdauungs- und N-Bilanzversuch an 12 Ferkeln (65.–80. Lebenstag) sowie bilanzierte Futtermischungen mit einem Austausch von bis zu 30 Prozent Weizen gegen teilentschälte Gerste im Wachstumstest ($n = 48$, 42.–100. Lebenstag) geprüft. Das Teilentschälen (Verminderung des Rohfasergehaltes von 5,9 auf 4,6 % der TS) führte zu folgenden *relativen* Veränderungen:

- Anstieg der Rohproteinverdaulichkeit um 1 %
- Anstieg der Rohkohlehydratverdaulichkeit um 3,7 %
- Anstieg der Energiekonzentration um 5 %
- Anstieg der Lysinwirksamkeit um 6,7 %
- Rückgang der Proteinqualität infolge verminderter Lysinkonzentration um 5 %

Insgesamt bleiben beachtliche Differenzen zum Futterwert von Weizen beim Ferkel bestehen. Da in der verwendeten bilanzierten Futtermischung weder Energie- noch Lysingehalt leistungsbegrenzend wirkten, führte der Einsatz von bis zu 30 % teilentschälter Gerste zu keinem nachhaltigen Effekt im Wachstumstest.

Sektion Tierproduktion und Veterinärmedizin der Karl-Marx-Universität Leipzig, Wissenschaftbereich Tierernährungschemie, Jena

G. RICHTER, ANNELORE LEMSER, B. MEIXNER und K. GRUHN

Tapiokaeinsatz bei Geflügel

Mittels Differenzverfahren wurde an Legehennen für thailändisches Tapiokamehl eine scheinbare Verdaulichkeit der org. Subs. von 88,3 %, des Rohproteins von 50,4 %, des Rohfetts von 25,1 %, der Rohfaser von 12,7 % und der N-fr. E. von 94,2 % ermittelt. Mit jeweils einem Fütterungsversuch an Küken und Junghennen der Legerichtung bzw. an Mastputen wurden 5, 20 bzw. 30 % Tapiokamehl als Substituent für Getreide ohne Methioninzusatz geprüft. Im Küken- und Junghennenfutter sind bis zu 20 % Tapiokamehl ohne Leistungsminderung einsetzbar. In der Putenmast war bei Tapiokaeinsatz die Körpermassezunahme vermindert und der Futteraufwand erhöht. Deshalb erscheint Tapioka bei Mastputen ungeeignet. Bei Legehennen und Broilern wurden jeweils zwei Versuche mit 5–30 % Tapioka durchgeführt. Die Eiproduktion sank geringfügig bei 10 % und mehr Tapiokaanteil. Es wird deshalb eine Einsatzgrenze von 5 % empfohlen. Bei 20 % Tapioka betrug die Leistungsminderung 1,5 %, so daß bei preisgünstigem Tapiokaangebot auch 20 % Tapioka im Legehennenfutter ökonomisch sein können. Tapiokamehl vermindert die Gelbfärbung der Eidotter. In der Broilermast konnten 30 % Tapioka im Starter- und Mastfutter ohne Leistungsminderung eingesetzt werden. Aus Sicherheitsgründen wird bei Broilern eine Einsatzgrenze von 20 % vorgeschlagen.

Sektion Tierproduktion und Veterinärmedizin der Karl-Marx-Universität Leipzig, Wissenschaftsbereich Tierernährungschemie

K. Gruhn

Zum Futterwert von Abfallknochen

Im Verdauungsversuch mit 5 kolostomierten Leghorn-Hähnen erfolgte nach separater Prüfung der scheinbaren Verdaulichkeit der Rohnährstoffe, des Lysins und der Thioaminosäuren der Gerste die Bestimmung der scheinbaren Verdaulichkeit der gleichen Komponenten von Schweineknochenbrei nach dem Differenzverfahren. Der tägliche Verzehr je Hahn betrug 40 g Gerste (incl. Mineral- und Wirkstoffe) und 60 g Knochenbrei. In der folgenden Tabelle werden die analytischen Daten der Rohnährstoffe und Aminosäuren in g/kg Originalsubstanz und deren scheinbare Verdaulichkeit von Gerste und Knochenbrei mitgeteilt.

Parameter	Analysendaten		scheinbare Verdaulichkeit in %	
	Gerste	Knochen	Gerste	Knochen
Organische Substanz	838	206	84,0	78,7
Rohprotein	129	125	82,5	65,8
Rohfett	34	60	58,9	95,0
N-freie Extraktstoffe	639	22	88,9	92,1
Lysin	5,1	6,6	77,6	79,9
Thioaminosäuren	3,9	1,7	77,8	65,0

Der Rohprotein-, Rohfett- und Rohaschegehalt des Knochenbreies betrug in der Trockensubstanz 25,2 %, 12,0 % bzw. 58,3 %. Gleichzeitig auf der Grundlage von Produktionsexperimenten an Schweinen kann der Knochenbrei in einer Menge von 500 ... 750 g je Mastschwein und Tag gedämpft mit Sammelfutter oder Küchenabfällen oder im Gemisch mit anderen Futterkomponenten verabreicht werden.

Forschungszentrum für Tierproduktion Dummerstorf-Rostock der Akademie der Landwirtschaftswissenschaften der DDR, Bereich Tierernährung „Oskar Kellner"

W. Matzke und W. Kracht

Der Futterwert von Sudrückstand aus der Gelatineproduktion

Bei der Herstellung von Gelatine fallen beim Aussuden Rückstände an, die als Sudrückstand (SR) bezeichnet werden. Im Mittel von 46 Proben wurden je kg Originalsubstanz (OS) 120 g Trockensubstanz, 3 g Rohasche, 58 g Rohprotein, 56 g Rohfett und 3 g NFE ermittelt. Im SR-

Protein sind je 16 g N 4,52 g Lysin, 1,04 g Methionin und Zystin sowie 2,54 g Threonin enthalten. Im Fett des SR überwiegen folgende langkettige, ungesättigte bzw. gesättigte Fettsäuren: Ölsäure 39 %, Palmitinsäure 28 %, Stearinsäure 15 %. Die Verdaulichkeit der organischen Substanz betrug 89 %, die des Rohproteins 98 % und die des Rohfettes 70 %. Der EFs-Gehalt betrug 140/kg OS und der Gehalt an verdaulichem Rohprotein 57 g/kg OS. Der Futterwert der SR wurde in 3 Mastversuchen an insgesamt 732 Schweinen geprüft. Bei Verabreichung von 1,5, 2,0 oder 3,0 kg SR zu restriktiven Mischfuttergaben wurden Mehrzunahmen von 83, 85 und 104 g erzielt. Der Fettgehalt der Schlachtkörper war bei SR-Gaben über 2,0 kg erhöht. Es wird empfohlen, je Tier und Tag 1,5–2,0 kg SR zu verabreichen.

Forschungszentrum für Tierproduktion Dummerstorf-Rostock der Akademie der Landwirtschaftswissenschaften der DDR, Bereich Tierernährung „Oskar Kellner"

W. Kracht und W. Matkze

Untersuchungen zum Futterwert von ölhaltigen Bleicherden

Bei der Raffination von Speisefetten bzw. -ölen fallen fett- bzw. ölhaltige Bleicherden (ÖB) an, die sich je nach Art der verwendeten Filtertechnik in ihrer Zusammensetzung unterscheiden. Die bei der Verwendung konventioneller Rahmenfilterpressen anfallenden (ÖBk) enthielten im Mittel von 56 Proben je kg Originalsubstanz (OS) 976 g Trockensubstanz (TS), 562 g Rohasche (RA), 261 g Rohfett (RF), 176 g N-freie Extraktstoffe (NFE). In der bei Verwendung von ZFS-Filtern anfallenden ÖB (ZFS) wurden im Mittel von 25 Proben je kg OS: 981 g TS, 618 g RA, 224 g RF und 149 g NFE ermittelt. Das Rohfett der ÖB enthielt vorwiegend langkettige und zu 85 % ungesättigte Fettsäuren, von denen die Erukasäure mit 31 %, die Ölsäure mit 24 % und die Linolsäure mit 20 % dominierten. In etwa 75 % der Proben wurden Peroxidzahlen von 20 ermittelt. In Verdauungsversuchen an Mastschweinen wurden bei Gaben von 200–300 g Verdaulichkeiten des Fettes von etwa 90 % und der NFE von 40–70 % ermittelt. Auf der Grundlage der Verdauungswerte wurden Nettoenergiegehalte von 644 (ÖBk) bzw. 550 (ÖB ZFS) EFs/kg OS errechnet. In 3 Mastversuchen an insgesamt 706 Schweinen wurde die Futterwirkung der ÖB (k) und (ZFS) geprüft.

Bei Substitution von Alleinfutter durch ÖB wurden Depressionen erzielt. Bei der Zulage der ÖB zu restriktiv verabreichten Alleinfutterrationen war ebenfalls kein positiver Effekt sichtbar.

Die aus dem Anstieg des Linolsäuregehaltes im Rückenspeck erkennbare Einlagerung von ÖB-Fett im Tierkörper bewirkte, offenbar infolge anderer depressiv wirkender Faktoren, keine Verbesserung der Mastleistung.

Akademie der Landwirtschaftswissenschaften der DDR, Forschungszentrum für Tierproduktion Dummerstorf-Rostock, Bereich Tierernährung „Oskar Kellner"

U. Kesting

Futterwert und Einsatz von Grobfutter beim Schwein

Von einigen ausgewählten Grobfutterarten (Luzerne verschiedener Rohfaserstufen, Roggen, Rotklee, Lupinen, Mais) wurde der Umfang der präzäkalen scheinbaren Nährstoffverdaulichkeit und die fäkale Nährstoffverdaulichkeit an ilealfistulierten Sauen ermittelt. Im Durchschnitt der untersuchten Chargen wurde das Rohprotein präzäkal am höchsten verdaut. Grobfutterproben mit Rohfasergehalten über 25 % der TS wurden (mit Einschränkung für Rohprotein) vollständig im Dickdarm fermentiert. Bei diesen Proben entsprach die gemessene fäkale Verdaulichkeit dem Umfang der Dickdarmfermentation. Unter Berücksichtigung der geringeren energetischen Ausbeute der

Dickdarmfermentation wird künftig ein gestaffelter Abzug der berechneten Energiekonzentration auf der Basis der verdaulichen Nährstoffe nach SCHIEMANN u. a. (1971) vorgenommen. Bei Grobfutterstoffen mit einem Rohfasergehalt unter 25 %, 25–28 %, und über 28 % beträgt der Abzug entsprechend 10, 15 und 20 %.

Im Vergleich zu Getreidemischungen, in denen die Dickdarmfermentation nur 10–15 % an der Gesamtverdauung ausmacht, sind Grobfutterstoffe für den Einsatz in der Mast ungeeignet. Sie haben bei Rationsanteilen zwischen 5 und 8 % nur diätetische Bedeutung. Für die Sauenfütterung sind Rationsanteile an Grobfutter bis zu 40 % vertretbar (güste und nieder tragende Tiere), wobei neben der guten diätetischen Wirkung auch das Grobfutterprotein für die AS-Versorgung zum Tragen kommt.

Forschungszentrum für Tierproduktion Dummerstorf-Rostock der Akademie der Landwirtschaftswissenschaften der DDR, Bereich Tierernährung „Oskar Kellner"

F. KREIENBRING und J. WÜNSCHE

Scheinbare präzäkale und fäkale Verdaulichkeit des Rohproteins und Resorption einiger Aminosäuren von Grobfuttermitteln beim Schwein

Die Untersuchungen erfolgten an ♀ Mastschweinen, die mit einer einfachen Ileumfistel ausgerüstet worden waren. In Zulageversuchen wurden 8 Luzerneproben (verschiedene Schnittzeiten nach technischer Trocknung sowie je eine frische, gefrostete, getrocknete oder silierte Probe gleichen Ausgangsmaterials) und getrocknete Proben von Futterroggen, Maisganzpflanzen und Rotklee auf die präzäkale und fäkale Verdaulichkeit des Rohproteins (sV-RP) und des Lys, Met, Cys, Thr, Try unter Anwendung der salzsäureunlöslichen Asche als Marker untersucht. Die präzäkale sV-RP erreichte bei allen Grobfuttermitteln maximal 48 %. Besonders stark beeinträchtigt war die präzäkale Resorption von Lys und Cys; dabei ergibt sich eine gesicherte positive Beziehung zwischen Lysingehalt des RP der Luzerneproben und seiner scheinbaren Resorption. Die Bakterientätigkeit im Dickdarm bewirkt, daß die am Ende des Ileums vorhandenen Verdaulichkeits-/Resorptionsunterschiede im Kot nicht mehr sichtbar sind. Wegen des stark eingeschränkten AS-Lieferungsvermögens ist aus der Sicht der Proteinbewertung ein Einsatz von Grobfuttermitteln in der Mast nicht zu empfehlen.

Sektion Tierproduktion der Wilhelm-Pieck-Universität Rostock, Wissenschaftsbereich Tierernährung

W. WIESEMÜLLER, K. MÜLLER und S. POPPE

Untersuchungen zum Futterwert von Luzerneblatt

Luzerne wurde bei einer Wuchshöhe von 50 cm mit 3 L H_2SO_4/t Grünmasse im Feldbestand behandelt. Nach 3 Tagen Sikkation wurde das Blatt mit einer Spezialmaschine separat geerntet und siliert. Die Silage hatte einen pH-Wert von 3,8 und war buttersäurefrei. Sie wurde an 185 kg schweren ileal fistulierten Sauen (Indikator HCl-unlösliche Asche) im Verdauungsversuch geprüft:

	Ausgangs-material	Silage	Verdaulichkeit aus Silage (%) scheinb. fäkal	scheinb. ileal	wahr ileal
Org. Substanz	890 g/kg TS	887 g/kg TS	64,4	41,6	–
Rohfaser	167 g/kg TS	178 g/kg TS			
Rohprotein	310 g/kg TS	272 g/kg TS	72,8	56,0	–
davon pl*	58,0 %	75,7 %			
Lysin		5,8 g/100 g RP	80,2	69,1	78,2
davon pl		73,5 %			

* pl = Pepsin-HCl-löslich

Nur zwei Drittel der org. Substanz werden ileal verdaut.

Forschungszentrum für Tierproduktion Dummerstorf-Rostock der Akademie der Landwirtschaftswissenschaften der DDR, Bereich Tierernährung „Oskar Kellner“

W. KRACHT und W. MATZKE

Futterwert und Einsatz von Rüben bei Schweinen

Zucker- (ZR) und Futterzuckerrüben (FZR) werden von Mastschweinen häufig nicht in ausreichendem Maße verzehrt, so daß die Mastleistungen nicht befriedigen. In unseren Mastversuchen wurde die Auswirkung des Waschens der Rüben im Vergleich zum Trockenreinigen, die Auswirkung des Zwischenlagerns zerkleinerter Rüben vor der Fütterung, der Effekt des Dämpfens und die Silierung mit einem Anteil von 8 % Rapsextraktionsschrot (RES) untersucht. Beim Anbau auf schwerem Boden ist das Waschen unerläßlich, die häufig übliche Zwischenlagerung über mehrere Tage führt zu Nährstoffverlusten und Leistungsdepressionen. Erste Befunde zum Dämpfeffekt zeigen, daß durch Dämpfen der FZR eine Verzehrs- und Leistungssteigerung erreichbar ist, während bei ZR nur eine geringe Wirkung vorlag. Bei Fütterung einer Silage aus ZR mit 8 % RES wurden hohe Mastleistungen erzielt.

Sektion Tierproduktion und Veterinärmedizin der Karl-Marx-Universität Leipzig, Wissenschaftsbereich Tierernährungsphysiologie und Futtermittelkunde [1]
LPG „Paul Fröhlich“ Leipzig, Versuchsabteilung [2]
Sektion Pflanzenproduktion der Martin-Luther-Universität Halle–Wittenberg, Lehrstuhl Ackerfutter [3]

H. JEROCH [1], SIGRUN SOUFFRANT [2] und W. RÖTSCHKE [3]

Futterwert von Restmais

Nach der fraktionierten Ernte von Maiskolben zur Gewinnung von Maiskorn-Spindel-Gemisch im Rahmen des Pflückdruschverfahrens verbleibt eine nicht unwesentliche Menge an Pflanzensubstanz auf dem Feld. Diese besteht aus stehengebliebenen Stengelteilen, meist bis zur Höhe der Kolbenansatzstelle (60 ... 90 cm) sowie Stengelspitzen, Blattspreiten, Lieschblättern, Kolbenstielen und größeren Spindelteilen. Für die Ernte des Restmaises steht derzeitig der Feldhäcksler E 280 bzw. E 281 mit dem Schlegeladapter „Orkan 89“ zur Verfügung. Nach diesem Verfahren geernteter Restmais weist folgenden mittleren Rohnährstoffgehalt (je kg TS) auf: 74 g Rohprotein, 300 g Rohfaser, 143 g Rohasche, 9 g Rohfett, 474 g N-freie Extraktstoffe. Der Rohaschegehalt ist durch verfahrensbedingte Erdbeimengungen gegenüber Restmais mittels Handernte um 50 % erhöht. Mit Hammeln durchgeführte Verdaulichkeitsmessungen ergaben folgendes Ergebnis: Org. Subst. 62 %, Energie 58 %, Rohprotein 16 %, Rohfaser 72 %, Rohfett 32 %, N-freie Extraktstoffe 61 %. Auf der Grundlage der gemessenen Verdaulichkeiten wurden 437 EFr und 12 g verdauliches Rohprotein je kg Restmaistrockensubstanz berechnet. Der energetische Futterwert von Restmais entspricht etwa dem von mittlerem Wiesenheu.

Sektion Tierproduktion und Veterinärmedizin der Karl-Marx-Universität Leipzig, Wissenschaftsbereich Tierernährungsphysiologie und Futtermittelkunde

C. Wecke, H. Jeroch und G. Gebhardt

Einsatz von Silosickersaft bei Mastschweinen

In Einzelfütterungsversuchen an Mastschweinen wurde geprüft, ob sich Silosickersaft (≈7 % Trockensubstanz) von Rübenblattsilage auf Grund seines relativ hohen Rohproteingehaltes (230–300 g/kg TS) eignet, herkömmliche Eiweißfuttermittel partiell zu ersetzen. Der Austausch von durchschnittlich 13 % des Eiweißkonzentrates in einer Ration mit CCM-Silage gegen Silosickersaft wirkte sich nicht nachteilig auf den Futterverzehr aus. Die Zunahmen waren nur geringfügig vermindert (um 2 %). Der Energie- und Rohproteinaufwand erhöhte sich mit dem Silosickersafteinsatz um 6 bzw. 3 % und die Schlachtkörperqualität wurde in der Tendenz verschlechtert. Die Einsparung von etwa 3,5 kg Eiweißkonzentrat pro Tier und Mastperiode war also nur auf Kosten einer ungünstigeren Futterökonomie möglich. Silosickersaft von Rübenblattsilage ist demnach nicht geeignet, proteinreiche Konzentrate in der Mastschweinefütterung zu substituieren.

Sektion Tierproduktion und Veterinärmedizin der Karl-Marx-Universität Leipzig, Wissenschaftsbereich Tierernährungschemie, Jena

G. Richter, H.-J. Löhnert, G. Flachowsky und J. Schwartze

Untersuchungen zum Futterwert von Chicoreewurzeln

Zur besseren Beurteilung des Futterwertes von getriebenen Chicoreewurzeln, dem Abfallprodukt der Chicoreeproduktion, wurden Verdauungsversuche mit je 5 Hammeln durchgeführt. Der Trockensubstanzgehalt der Wurzeln betrug lediglich 125 g/kg Frischmasse; je kg Trockensubstanz waren 810 g Rohkohlenhydrate enthalten. Für die Verdaulichkeit der org. Subst. der getriebenen Chicoreewurzeln wurden 84 %, für die Energiekonzentration 630 EFr/kg TS ermittelt. Getriebene Chicoreewurzeln sollten gewaschen an Schafe und Mastrinder (≈2 kg Frischmasse/100 kg Lebendmasse und Tag), aber nicht an Milchkühe gefüttert werden.

Institut für Futterproduktion Paulinenaue der Akademie der Landwirtschaftswissenschaften der DDR

O. Knabe, K.-D. Robowsky, R. Schuppenies und G. Weise

Qualitätsmerkmale und Futterwert von Maissilagen

Der TS-Gehalt des entlieschten Kolbens ist ein wesentliches Merkmal für die Beurteilung des Nährstoffgehaltes und der Energiekonzentration (EK). Erntereifer Silomais hat einen TS-Gehalt im Kolben von 35–45 % (Lieschkolben = 30–40 %; Gesamtpflanze = 24–30 %). Steigender TS-

Gehalt bewirkt eine Abnahme des Rohfasergehaltes und den Anstieg des Stärkegehaltes und der EK bis zu einem TS-Gehalt im Kolben von 35 %. Bei weiterem Anstieg des TS-Gehaltes treten nur noch unbedeutende Veränderungen ein. Zwischen getrockneten und silierten Ganzpflanzen von gleichem erntereifem Ausgangsmaterial bestehen nur geringe Unterschiede in der EK. Für die Bewertung von Siliergut und Maissilagen können gleiche Werte unterstellt werden.

Gärintensität und Silierverluste nehmen mit steigendem TS-Gehalt des Siliergutes ab. Der WKH-Anteil wird nahezu vollständig vergoren. Der Umfang der Stärkevergärung ist vom TS-Gehalt und vom Kolbenanteil abhängig.

Der Stärkegehalt ist nicht für die Kennzeichnung der EK, des TS-Gehaltes oder des Kolbenanteiles geeignet.

Für die Qualitätsbewertung von Maissilagen werden in Zusammenhang mit einer neuen Schätzgleichung veränderte Qualitätsparameter wirksam. Eine Verbindlichkeit wird für die Ernte 87/88 angestrebt.

Institut für Futterproduktion Paulinenaue der Akademie der Landwirtschaftswissenschaften der DDR

W. Seyfarth, O. Knabe und G. Weise

Eiweißabbau während des Welkens von Grünfutterstoffen

Die Proteolyse ist durch Welken nicht zu unterbinden. Sie setzt durch Tätigkeit pflanzeneigener Enzyme sofort nach dem Schnitt ein und läßt sich durch exogene Faktoren nicht oder kaum verhindern.

In Abhängigkeit von der Liegezeit und damit auch vom Massebelag tritt ein Verlust an Reinprotein (Gräser >25 %, Luzerne >17 %) und einzelnen Aminosäuren auf. Bei Gräsern verminderte sich der Rohproteinanteil am Rohprotein bei günstiger Witterung um ca. 15 % (2 kg/m^2) bis 20 % (6 kg/m^2), bei ungünstiger Witterung um ca. 30 % (unabhängig vom Massebelag). Bei Luzerne sank der Reinproteinanteil um 7–10 %.

Bis zu 35 % ihres Ausgangswertes nahmen beim Welken ab: Ala, Lys, Glu, Gly, Arg, Leu und Tyr; der Pro-Gehalt erhöhte sich bis um 140 %.

Bei Luzerne wurde Met vollständig abgebaut.

Im Welkgut (Gräser, Luzerne) bildeten sich z. T. bereits Essigsäure und Äthanol.

Bei hohen Werten für Lufttemperatur und bei kurzen Feldliegezeiten war der Lys-Abbau geringer als bei kühlem, feuchten Wetter (Abnahme des Lys-Gehaltes unabhängig vom Massebelag bis zu 42,5 % des Ausgangswertes).

Kurze Feldliegezeiten und geringe Massebeläge (Breitablage) vermindern die Desmolyse (Ausnahme: Lys) und schränken die Proteolyse ein.

Institut für Futterproduktion Paulinenaue der Akademie der Landwirtschaftswissenschaften der DDR

W. Seyfarth, O. Knabe und G. Weise

Eiweißabbau während der Silierung von Grünfutterstoffen

Der Reinproteingehalt der Gräser verringert sich bei anaerober Silierung auf 60–70 % des Ausgangswertes, wobei der Reinproteinabbau mit dem TS-Gehalt des Einlagerungsgutes negativ korreliert. Bei anaerober Frisch- und Welksilierung stellt sich ein konstantes Reinprotein-NPN-Verhältnis von etwa 40 : 60 % in der Silage ein.

Bei Frischsilierung von Gräsern mit schlechter Siliereignung und ohne wirksamen Siliermittelzusatz treten Reinprotein- und Gesamtaminosäureverluste bis zu 60 % auf. Mit steigendem TS-Gehalt wird die Desaminierung der Aminosäuren gehemmt.
Bei anaerober Frischsilierung von Rübenblatt sinkt der Reinproteingehalt auf ca. 70 % des Ausgangswertes.

Auch in buttersäurefreien Silagen sind beträchtliche Änderungen im Gehalt an einzelnen Aminosäuren bei annähernder Konstanz des Gesamtaminosäuregehaltes zu erwarten.

Als Indikatoren für desmolytische Abbaureaktionen traten auf:
γ-Aminovaleriansäure, α-Aminobuttersäure, Ornithin, Diaminopimelinsäure, Galaktosamin, Glukosamin (>2 mg/g TS)

Die desmolytischen Abbauprozesse werden durch Lufteinfluß verstärkt.

Institut für Futterproduktion Paulinenaue der Akademie der Landwirtschaftswissenschaften der DDR

P. Lepom und Helga Kloss

Bildung von Sterigmatocystin auf Grobfutter durch Aspergillus versicolor

Es wurden 69 Grobfutterproben aus der landwirtschaftlichen Praxis auf den Befall mit A. versicolor untersucht, in denen der Pilz mit einer Stetigkeit von 14,5 % vorkam. Die von Grobfutter isolierten A. versicolor-Stämme wurden unter in vitro-Bedingungen auf ihr Sterigmatocystinbildungsvermögen getestet.

Alle Isolate bildeten auf Mais Sterigmatocystin; dagegen war das Toxinbildungsvermögen auf Heu und Stroh vergleichsweise gering. Auf der Basis der durchgeführten Untersuchungen wird die Wahrscheinlichkeit eines natürlichen Vorkommens von Sterigmatocystin in Stroh und Heu in toxikologisch relevanten Konzentrationen als relativ gering eingeschätzt. Zur weiteren Absicherung der Ergebnisse sind gezielte Untersuchungen zum Vorkommen von Sterigmatocystin in makroskopisch mit Schimmel befallenen Grobfutterpartien dringend erforderlich.

Forschungszentrum für Tierproduktion Dummerstorf-Rostock der Akademie der Landwirtschaftswissenschaften der DDR,
Bereich Tierernährung „Oskar Kellner“

U. Herrmann, J. Wünsche, Marlis Meinl und U. Hennig

Untersuchungen zur Aminosäurenresorption pflanzlicher proteinreicher Futtermittel beim Schwein

An intakten sowie mit Ileorektal-Anastomosen versehenen Schweinen wurden die scheinbare Rohproteinverdaulichkeit (sV-RP) und scheinbare Aminosäurenresorption (sR-AS) im Gesamttrakt (ges) bzw. präzäkal am Dünndarmende (pz) von Sojaextraktionsschrot (SES), Ackerbohnen (AB) und gelben Süßlupinen (Lu), deren Rationsanteile 200, 308 bzw. 216 g/kg TS betrugen, mittels Differenzverfahren bestimmt. Geprüft wurde der Einfluß eines unterschiedlich starken Zerkleinerungsgrades dieser Futtermittel. In den Varianten „grob“ waren bei SES, AB und Lu 18, 19 bzw. 16 % der Partikel >2 mm und in allen Varianten „fein“ nahezu 100 % <2 mm. Zwischen den Behandlungsvarianten ergaben sich sowohl pz als auch ges für die sV-RP und sR-AS keine signifikanten Unterschiede. Die sV-RP ist pz etwa 10 Einheiten signifikant niedriger als ges, stellt aber – ebenso wie die pz sR-AS – das bessere Kriterium zur Beurteilung der Proteinqualität dar.

Forschungszentrum für Tierproduktion Dummerstorf-Rostock der Akademie der Landwirtschaftswissenschaften der DDR,
Bereich Tierernährung „Oskar Kellner“

K. KRAWIELITZKI, RUTHILD SCHADEREIT und BRIGITTA EVERS

Bestimmung von Darmpassage und N-Verdaulichkeit bei Ratten unter Verwendung von $^{51}Cr_2O_3$ und TiO_2 als Marker

Die Passage beider Marker durch Magen, Duodenum, Jejunum und Ileum erfolgt nach einmaliger Gabe kontinuierlich (9,1 ±0,3 % der verabfolgten Menge pro Stunde). Die Markerausscheidung im Kot beginnt in Abhängigkeit vom Rohfasergehalt 8 h (RFa = 5,1 % d. TS) bzw. 5 h (RFa = 9,4 % d. TS) nach der Verabfolgung und ist nach 2 ... 3 Tagen beendet. Ein Vergleich der Passagezeit verschiedener Futtermittel wird bei 50 % Markerausscheidung empfohlen.

Die Werte für die N-Verdaulichkeit nach der konventionellen Methode und nach der Indikatormethode unter Verwendung von $^{51}Cr_2O_3$ bzw. TiO_2 als Marker sind praktisch gleich. Die Indikatormethode ist unabhängig von etwaigen Futter- bzw. Kotverlusten. Sie ist mit geringeren Probenmengen durchführbar und erübrigt Sammelproben über mehrere Tage.

Die Indikatormethode mit $^{51}Cr_2O_3$ oder TiO_2 liefert daher zuverlässigere Werte für die N-Verdaulichkeit als die konventionelle Methode.

Beide Marker sind für die Bestimmung der Passagezeit und der N-Verdaulichkeit bei Ratten geeignet.

Sektion Tierproduktion und Veterinärmedizin der Karl-Marx-Universität Leipzig, Wissenschaftsbereich Tierernährungsphysiologie und Futtermittelkunde

INGRID HALLE und G. GEBHARDT

Prüfung von Fertigfutter an Hunden und Katzen

In längerfristigen Versuchen wurden vollwertige, pelletierte Alleinfutter an Welpen, wachsenden und ausgewachsenen Hunden und Katzen sowie Zuchttieren geprüft. Die Versuchsfuttermischungen wurden aus volkswirtschaftlich verfügbaren Rohstoffen unter Berücksichtigung der Bedarfsansprüche der Tiere zusammengestellt. Als Kontrollfutter fand jeweils ein international geprüftes Alleinfutter Verwendung. In der Futter-, Rohprotein- und Energieaufnahme sowie bei den Körpermasseveränderungen traten zwischen Versuchs- und Kontrollgruppen keine signifikanten Unterschiede auf. Die Akzeptanz der Futtermischungen war gut und beide Tierarten verzehrten bedarfsdeckende Mengen. Schlußfolgernd aus den Untersuchungen wurde festgestellt, daß die Fütterung der neuentwickelten, trockenen Alleinfutter an Hunden und Katzen verschieden Alters möglich ist.

Sektion Tierproduktion und Veterinärmedizin der Karl-Marx-Universität Leipzig, Wissenschaftsbereich Tierernährungschemie, Jena

F. SCHÖNE, KIRSTEN PORZIG, H. LÜDKE und J. BRYS

Beeinflussung der Leistung der Ferkel nach dem Absetzen durch Futterzusammensetzung, Ergotropikaeinsatz sowie Absetzmasse

In einem dreifaktoriellen Versuch wurde neben üblichem Ferkelaufzuchtfutter mit 20 % Rohprotein (RP) (Standard), eine energiereiche und eine proteinarme (16 % RP) Diät an 216 gleichaltrigen (33 ±4 d) aber unterschiedlich schweren Ferkeln (Absetzmasse 5,5 bis 9 kg) geprüft. Die drei Rationen in drei Absetzmasseklassen wurden über 21 d jeweils ohne und mit Bisergon gefüttert. Vom 22. bis 71. d nach dem Absetzen erhielten die Ferkel einheitlich die Standarddiät ohne Ergotropikum.

Die Mehrzunahme durch den Bisergonzusatz variierte von 9 % bei den schweren energiereich bis zu 150 % bei den leichten proteinarm ernährten Ferkeln. Nach 10 Wochen waren die mit Bisergon gestarteten Tiere ($\bar{x}$ 34,6 kg) signifikant schwerer als die Kontrolltiere ($\bar{x}$ 31,6 kg). Bei proteinarmer Ernährung gelang es die Magen- und Darmerkrankungen einzuschränken. Die so gestarteten Ferkel mit einer Absetzmasse $<$7,5 kg konnten aber von der 4. bis 10. Versuchswoche die Entwicklungsverzögerung nicht aufholen. Der Fetteinsatz für die Stabilisierung von Ferkeln $<$8 kg Absetzmasse sollte weiterhin untersucht werden.

Bezirksinstitut für Veterinärwesen Gera in Jena[1]
Sektion Tierproduktion und Veterinärmedizin der Karl-Marx-Universität Leipzig, Wissenschaftsbereich Tierernährungschemie, Jena[2]

U. LOBER[1], D. GEINITZ[1], G. FLACHOWSKY[2] und W. I. OCHRIMENKO[2]

Zur Wirkung von Niazin in der Futterration auf einige Stoffwechsel- und Leistungskriterien frischlaktierender Kühe

In einem Praxisversuch wurden 14 an subklinischer Ketose erkrankte, frischlaktierende Kühe so in 2 Gruppen zusammengestellt, daß zu Versuchsbeginn nahezu identische ketogene Belastung und Milchleistung gegeben waren.

Bei gleichem nicht bedarfsdeckendem Ernährungsregime (11,9 kg TS; 5,9 kEFr und 710 g vRP bei 18 kg Milchleistung je Kuh und Tag) erhielten die Versuchskühe über einen Zeitraum von 30 Tagen täglich 10 g Niazin, verteilt auf 2 Futterzeiten. Am 3., 7., 14., 21. und 28. Tag wurden Blutproben durch Vena-jugularis-Punktion gewonnen und auf die Parameter β-Hydroxybuttersäure (β-OHBS), Glukose und Harnstoff (nur 21. und 28. Tag) untersucht. Vor dem Versuchsbeginn und im Abstand von 4 Wochen wurden insgesamt 5mal die Milchmenge und der Milchfettgehalt ermittelt.

Die Niazinzulage erbrachte eine Verminderung der β-OHBS-Konzentration im Blutserum um 45 % bis zum 7. Versuchstag, verminderte Blut-Harnstoff-Werte, tendenziell höhere Blut-Glukose-Konzentrationen, Steigerung der Milchmenge um 2,6 %, Erhöhung des Milchfettgehaltes um 3,8 % und eine bessere Persistenz der Laktationskurve.

Es wird vorgeschlagen, Niazin in der landwirtschaftlichen Praxis für frischlaktierende, leistungsfähige Kühe zu nutzen und weitere Untersuchungen zu spezifischen Niazinwirkungen durchzuführen.

Sektion Tierproduktion und Veterinärmedizin der Karl-Marx-Universität Leipzig, Wissenschaftsbereich Tierernährungschemie, Jena[1] und Wissenschaftsbereich Tieranatomie, Tierhistologie und Embryologie, Leipzig[2]

BRIGITTA KIRSCHE, M. SCHLENZIG, W. I. OCHRIMENKO, G. FLACHOWSKY, G. MICHEL[2] und A. HENNIG

Einfluß abgestufter β-Karotingaben auf den Karotingehalt verschiedener Fraktionen des Ovars von Jungrindern

An 32 Masthybridfärsen wurde über 120 Tage eine karotinarme Stroh-Konzentrat-Ration (Karotingehalt: $<$1 mg/kg TS) gefüttert. Neben 10000 IE Vitamin A je 100 kg Lebendmasse und Tag erhielten je 8 Jungrinder keine Karotinergänzung bzw. 100, 200 oder 300 mg β-Karotin je Tier und Tag. Im zweiten Trächtigkeitsmonat erfolgte die Schlachtung der Färsen und die Ermittlung des β-Karotingehaltes in verschiedenen Fraktionen des Ovars.

Neben dem Corpus luteum wurde auch in orangefarbenen Gewebeeinschlüssen im Ovar Karotin gefunden. In beiden Fraktionen stieg die Karotinkonzentration mit zunehmender Karotinsupplementation an, wobei in den Gewebeeinschlüssen signifikant höhere Konzentrationen als im Corpus luteum gefunden wurden:

Parameter	β-Karotin-Supplementation (mg/Tier und Tag) 0	100	200	300
Masse des Corpus luteum (g)	4,3	4,5	3,8	4,6
Masse der Gewebeeinschlüsse (g)	0,19	0,25	0,43	0,36
Karotinkonzentration im Corpus luteum (μg/g)	2,3	27	50	81
Karotinkonzentration in Gewebeeinschlüssen (μg/g)	158	150	334	487

Sektion Tierproduktion und Veterinärmedizin der Karl-Marx-Universität Leipzig, Wissenschaftsbereich Tierernährungschemie, Jena

G. Flachowsky, Maria Matthey, M. Schneider und W. I. Ochrimenko

Bedeutung von Isosäuren für die Wiederkäuerernährung

Zu Isosäuren werden die verzweigtkettigen Fettsäuren Isobuttersäure, Isovaleriansäure und 2-Methylbuttersäure sowie Valeriansäure als lineare Fettsäurekette zusammengefaßt. Isosäuren entstehen im Pansen vor allem beim Abbau verzweigtkettiger Aminosäuren, wie z. B. Valin, Leuzin und Isoleuzin. Verschiedene Pansenmikroben benötigen die C-Gerüste der Isosäuren zur Synthese der entsprechenden Aminosäuren und damit für die mikrobielle Proteinerzeugung sowie für eine hohe zellulolytische Aktivität. In den vorliegenden Untersuchungen stieg mit zunehmendem Gehalt der Ration an nativem Protein die Konzentration der Isosäuren im Pansensaft an. Proteinherkunft, Höhe der Futtergabe und Energiegehalt der Ration üben ebenfalls Einfluß auf die Isosäurenkonzentration aus. Während bei konzentratreicher Rationsgestaltung (60 % Konzentrat) absolute und molare Konzentration der Isosäuren im Pansensaft nach der Fütterung anstiegen (von 0,37 auf 0,56 mmol/100 ml) bzw. annähernd konstant blieben (4,0–4,9 Mol %), fielen sie bei grobfutterreicher Ration (100 % Trockengrün) von 0,35 mmol/100 ml bzw. 5,5 Mol % vor der Fütterung auf 0,22 mmol/100 ml bzw. 2,4 Mol % 6 Stunden nach der Fütterung ab und stiegen dann allmählich wieder an.

Durch intraruminale Verabreichung eines Isosäurengemisches (2×1 g/kg TS und Tag, bestehend aus je 25 % Isobuttersäure, Isovaleriansäure, 2-Methylbuttersäure und Valeriansäure) zu einer Stroh-Stärke-Harnstoff-Ration (1000; 300 bzw. 50 g/Tier und Tag), stieg der Nylonbeutel-Trockensubstanzverlust von NH_3-behandeltem Stroh nach 48 h Inkubationszeit von 47 auf 49 % ($\alpha > 0{,}05$) an.

Weitere Untersuchungen über die Zweckmäßigkeit einer Isosäurensupplementation bei verschiedenen Rationen erscheinen zweckmäßig.

Sektion Tierproduktion und Veterinärmedizin der Karl-Marx-Universität Leipzig, Wissenschaftsbereich Tierernährungschemie, Jena

G. Richter, W. I. Ochrimenko, D. Geinitz, G. Flachowsky und A. Hennig

Untersuchungen zur Nutzung einheimischer Mineralstoffquellen (Mg; Co)

In 3 Bilanzversuchen mit Hammeln, 5 Mineralstoffaufnahmeversuchen mit wachsenden Jungrindern und einem Einzelfütterungsversuch mit Mastlämmern sollten Aussagen zur Eignung von Kieserit ($MgSO_4 \times H_2O$; 76 TGL 6442; 15,8 % Mg) bzw. Kobaltsulfat V 125 (12,5 % Co) als neue

Mg- bzw. Co-Träger für die Mineralstoffmischungen für Rinder gewonnen werden. Die Höhe der ermittelten scheinbaren Mg-Verdaulichkeit des Kieserits variierte in Abhängigkeit von Mg-Verarmung und der Mg-Aufnahme von ≈43 % bis 69 %. Durch den Kieseritzusatz in verschiedenen Mineralstoffmischungen für Rinder anstelle von kalziniertem $MgSO_4$ wurde unter Weidebedingungen die Aufnahme positiv beeinflußt.

In dem durchgeführten Mastlämmerversuch hatte das geprüfte Kobaltsulfat V 125 die gleiche Wirkung, wie das bisher in den Mineralstoffmischungen eingesetzte Kobaltsulfat I 206. Nach achtwöchiger Supplementation von 10 mg Co je Tier und Tag betrug die mittlere Co-Konzentration in der Leber 1,31 bzw. 1,42 mg/kg TS und die relative Co-Wiederfindungsrate des im Versuchszeitraum aufgenommenen Co betrug 0,03 bzw. 0,04 %

Sektion Tierproduktion und Veterinärmedizin der Karl-Marx-Universität Leipzig, Wissenschaftsbereich Tierernährungschemie, Jena

H. Lüdke, F. Schöne und K. Gruhn

Untersuchungen zur Phosphorversorgung von Absetzferkeln und Mastschweinen

Im Versuch I (Einzeltierhaltung, 7 Tiere/Gruppe, Lebendmasseabschnitt 11–40 kg, Gesamtfutterverzehr/Schwein 68 kg) untersuchten wir die Auswirkung einer Phosphor (P) Unterversorgung auf die Mastleistung sowie auf den Protein-, Fett-, Asche- und Phosphorgehalt der Weichgewebe und des Skelettes. Der P-Gehalt der Grundration betrug 2,97 g, die P-Zulage 2,5 g/kg Futter. Futterverzehr und Lebendmassezunahmen der P-unterversorgten Schweine waren um 13 bzw. 44 % geringer, der Futteraufwand um 60 % höher als bei ausreichender P-Versorgung.

Der Proteingehalt des Weichgewebehomogenates war um 11 % vermindert, der Fettgehalt um 36 % erhöht.

Im Versuch II (Gruppenhaltung, 20 Tiere/Gruppe, Lebendmasseabschnitt 26–120 kg) wurde der Einfluß einer P-Zulage von 1,5 g/kg zu zwei unterschiedlichen Rationen (Mais-Sojaextraktionsschrot; P-Gehalt 5,15 g/kg bzw. Gerste, Roggen, verschiedene Extraktionsschrote; P-Gehalt 5,28 g/kg) geprüft. Trotz hoher Tageszunahmen (>720 g) hatte die P-Zulage keinen Einfluß auf die Mastleistungsparameter. Der Aschegehalt in der Rippen-TS betrug unabhängig von der P-Zulage 48 % bei den Tieren, die die erste und 49 % bei denen, die die zweite Ration erhalten hatten.

Sektion Tierproduktion und Veterinärmedizin der Karl-Marx-Universität Leipzig, Wissenschaftsbereich Tierernährungschemie, Jena

B. Meixner

Möglichkeiten und Grenzen des Einsatzes örtlicher Futterreserven in der Broilermast

In einem 52tägigen Mastversuch wurden die Möglichkeiten des Einsatzes von Eiweißmischsilage, Futterquark und gedämpften Kartoffeln im partiellen Austausch von Broilermastalleinfutter untersucht. Der verminderte Trockensubstanzgehalt der Ration führte zur Steigerung der Futteraufnahme bis zu 70 %. Dadurch nahmen die Broiler die Nährstoffe annähernd bedarfsgerecht auf. Broilermastalleinfutter kann zu 50 % durch ≈10 % Eiweißmischsilage oder ≈10 % Futterquark in Verbindung mit Weizenschrot bei etwa gleichen Mastergebnissen ersetzt werden. Dem bis 40 % gesteigerten Futteraufwand steht ein dem Broilermastalleinfutter adäquater Rohprotein- und um 10 % erhöhter EF^{h}-Aufwand gegenüber. Gaben an gedämpften Kartoffeln über 20 % zum Broilermastalleinfutter führen nur bei gleichzeitigen Zulagen an Eiweißkonzentraten zu akzeptablen Mastleistungen. Die geprüften Futtermittel sollten erst ab 14. Masttag verabreicht werden, um Schnabelverklebungen, erhöhten Futterverlusten und damit verbundener Verunreinigung des Stalles vorzubeugen. Weitere Vorbedingungen sind geeignete Fütterungseinrichtungen für feuchtkrümeliges Futter, welche die wechselnden Trockensubstanzgehalte und die leichte Verderblichkeit derartiger Futterrationen berücksichtigen.

Sektion Tierproduktion und Veterinärmedizin der Karl-Marx-Universität Leipzig, Wissenschaftsbereich Tierfütterung und Ernährungsschäden

H. Schirmbeck, M. Hoffmann und A. Dittrich

Effektive Fütterungsregimes für die Aufzucht weiblicher Jungschafe

Weibliche Jungschafe der Rasse Merinofleischschaf wurden in 3 Einzelfütterungsversuchen (3. bis 6. und 7.–13. Lebensmonat) sowie in Gruppenfütterungsversuchen (7.–12. Lebensmonat) mit unterschiedlicher Intensität (mittel [m] = 100–130 g LMZ/d; hoch [h] > 130 g LMZ/d aufgezogen. Die Einzelfütterungsversuche enthielten nacheinander die Varianten m/h, m/m, h/m, h/h, die Gruppenfütterungsversuche die Varianten m oder h durchgängig. Die Trockensubstanzaufnahme (je Tier und Tag) war bei h/h 1156 g, h/m 1074 g, m/h 1060 g, m/m 1022 g und insgesamt bei h größer m. Dabei war die Aufnahme aus Gobfutterstoffen (je Tier und Tag) bei m/m 605 g, h/m 542 g, m/h 332 g, h/h 275 g. Im Alter von 12 bzw. 13 Lebensmonaten unterschieden sich die Lebendmassen signifikant, und zwar bei Einzelfütterung m/m 53,6 kg, m/h 60,3 kg, h/m 57,2 kg, h/h 63,9 kg, bei Gruppenfütterung m 61,0 kg, h 64,7 kg.

In den Gruppenfütterungsversuchen konnten zum Zeitpunkt der ersten Zuchtbenutzung keine signifikanten Lebendmasseunterschiede mehr festgestellt werden (m 59,8 kg, h 60,2 kg). Der Reinwollzuwachs (je Tier und Tag) betrug bei m/m 11,3 g, m/h 12,7 g, h/m 11,9 g, h/h 14,1 g. Der Energieaufwand je kg Lebendmassezunahme war bei m/m > m/h > h/m > h/h sowie in den Gruppenfütterungsversuchen bei h > m. Der Energieaufwand aus Konzentraten je kg Lebendmassezunahme war bei h um 176 % höher als bei m. Für den Energieaufwand je kg Reinwollzuwachs waren zwischen den Aufzuchtvarianten keine signifikanten Unterschiede feststellbar.

Sektion Tierproduktion und Veterinärmedizin der Humboldt-Universität zu Berlin, Bereich Sozialistische Betriebswirtschaft

Christa Brunsch und S. Jahn

Einfluß der Fütterung auf den Milcheiweißgehalt und ökonomische Auswirkungen

Ausgehend von der Aufgabenstellung, die Produktion von Hart-, Schnitt- und Weichkäse zu erhöhen, erfolgten in sechs Betrieben des Kreises Angermünde ökonomisch determinierte Untersuchungen zur Variabilität des Milcheiweißgehaltes.

Der wesentliche Einfluß auf den Milcheiweißgehalt geht von der Fütterung aus. Eine Erhöhung der Futterenergiezufuhr um 1 kEFr je Kuh und Tag bewirkte eine Steigerung des Milcheiweißgehaltes um 0,03 Prozent. Bei gleichbleibender Futterenergiezufuhr kann der Milcheiweißgehalt durch den gezielten Einsatz zuckerreicher Futtermittel positiv beeinflußt werden. Besondere Bemühungen um einen hohen Milcheiweißgehalt sind am Ende der Winterfütterungsperiode erforderlich. Parallel zu einem geringen Niveau der Futterenergiezufuhr lag der Eiweißgehalt im Monat April in allen Untersuchungsbetrieben um 0,08 bis 0,22 % unter dem Jahresdurchschnitt.

Als ökonomische Konsequenz verringerter Milcheiweißgehaltswerte sind ein erhöhter Grundmaterialverbrauch (0,23 bis 0,76 kg Milch mehr je kg Käse gegenüber dem Jahresdurchschnitt, für Tollenser mit 45 % Fett in der TS) und eine Senkung im wirtschaftlichen Ergebnis zu nennen.

Forschungszentrum für Tierproduktion Dummerstorf-Rostock der Akademie der Landwirtschaftswissenschaften der DDR, Bereich Tierernährung „Oskar Kellner“

K. Kolbitz und U. Grüner

Untersuchungen zum Konzentrataufwand in der Milchproduktion

Der leistungsfördernde Konzentrat (K)-Einsatz in der Milchproduktion ist eine wichtige Aufgabe bei der Entwicklung der Futterökonomie.

Als Ausgangspunkt für eine tiefgründige Analyse und für den Leistungsvergleich über die Entwicklung der Futterökonomie in der Milchproduktion wird zunächst für die Betriebe und Ställe bzw. Territorien die Höhe des K-Aufwandes/kg Milch in Abhängigkeit von der erreichten Milchleistung grafisch dargestellt. Grundlage der Einschätzung ist ein Abstandsvergleich zu einer allgemeinen K-Richtwertlinie, die auf der Basis des DDR-Futterbewertungssystems berechnet wurde. In der Tendenz wird folgendes sichtbar:

- Im Durchschnitt ist der K-Aufwand in der Milchproduktion noch zu hoch. Das deutet insbesondere auf eine ungenügende Ausnutzung des Grobfutteraufnahmevermögens der Kühe hin.
- Die Streuung der Einzelwerte sowohl hinsichtlich der Milchleistung als auch des K-Aufwandes (auch bei gleicher Leistung) ist beachtlich.
- Bei höheren Leistungen wird im allgemeinen der K-Richtwert durch die Betriebe besser eingehalten bzw. sogar unterboten. Damit werden futterökonomische Reserven für alle Betriebe angedeutet. Diese können jedoch nur durch eine tiefgründige Analyse im jeweiligen Betrieb erschlossen werden.

Zentralstelle für Futtermittelprüfung und Fütterung Halle-Lettin

J. Becker und W.-D. Schulze

Das Futtermittelregister der DDR – eingetragene Futtermittel und laufende Anträge

Nach den geltenden Bestimmungen, der Futtermittelverordnung (1964) und der Verordnung über Futterreserven (1984) sind alle Einzelfuttermittel, Mischfuttermittel, Wirk- und Mineralstoffmischungen, die keinem staatlichen Standard unterliegen, in das Futtermittelregister der DDR aufzunehmen, das die Zentralstelle für Futtermittelprüfung und Fütterung Halle-Lettin im Auftrag des Ministeriums für Land-, Forst- und Nahrungsgüterwirtschaft führt. Die Registrierung erfordert die Erfüllung bestimmter Voraussetzungen und verpflichtet den Hersteller zur Einhaltung der festgelegten Qualitätsparameter. Derzeitig sind im Futtermittelregister 25 Einzelfuttermittel und Mischungen erfaßt. Nach der Verordnung über die Gewinnung und Verwertung von Futterreserven sind die Produktions- und Aufkommensbetriebe verpflichtet, bisher noch nicht genutzte Futtermittel den Räten der Kreise zu melden. Gegenwärtig liegen Informationen zu 17 weiteren Produkten vor, über deren Eignung als Futtermittel nach entsprechender Prüfung zu entscheiden ist.

Forschungszentrum für Tierproduktion Dummerstorf-Rostock der Akademie der Landwirtschaftswissenschaften der DDR, Bereich Tierernährung „Oskar Kellner“

A. Chudy

Der Einsatz betriebsnaher Rechentechnik in den Landwirtschaftsbetrieben

Am Bürocomputer robotron A 5120/30 aus dem VEB Büromaschinenwerk Karl-Marx-Stadt wurden folgende im Betriebssystem SIOS 1526 in Assembler (MABS) erstellte Programme vorgeführt und erläutert:

1. „Berechnung komplexer Bedarfsnormen für Milchkühe (BEKUH)", das eine vom Laktationsverlauf abhängige Ermittlung der Bedarfsnormen einschl. Schätzung der Futteraufnahme ermöglicht, als Beispiel für künftig zu entwickelnde Programmmodule zur Bedarfsberechnung für alle Tierarten.
2. Rationsberechnung und Futtereinsatzplanung mit Angleichung der Rationen an einen vorgegebenen Futterfonds (RATBE II)
3. Planung und Bilanzierung von Futterbedarf und Futteraufkommen mit den Programmteilen zur Berechnung des Energie-, Nährstoff- und Naturalbedarfs (FUBED), zur Erfassung des Futteraufkommens (FUAUF), Futterbilanzierung (FUBIL) und zur Bilanzauswertung nach dem Prinzip der Fehl- und Austauschmengenrechnung (BILAU).

Forschungszentrum für Tierproduktion Dummerstorf-Rostock der Akademie der Landwirtschaftswissenschaften der DDR, Bereich Tierernährung „Oskar Kellner"

P. Grobbecker, R. Schiemann und L. Hoffmann

Zur Messung der motorischen Aktivität von Tieren in Respirationskammern

Es wurden Meßanordnungen zur kontinuierlichen Erfassung der motorischen Spontanaktivität (MSA) in Respirationskammern für Ratten und Schweine eingebaut mit dem Ziel, den Energiebedarf für MSA durch lineare Regression aus den minütlich abgespeicherten Daten der MSA und der Wärmeproduktion zu bestimmen. Für Ratten wurde ein optoelektronisches Meßverfahren gewählt, bei dem die Helligkeitsschwankungen des von der Tieroberfläche reflektierten Lichtes ausgewertet wurden, während die Aktivität beim Schwein mittels Kraftmeßdosen erfaßt wurde.

In Modellversuchen an Ratten (LM 80–100 g) wurde im Mittel aller 58 Versuchstage ein der MSA zuzuordnender Anteil der täglichen Wärmeproduktion von 12 ± 3 % ermittelt, während dieser Anteil bei Modellversuchen an Schweinen (LM 70–100 kg) im Mittel aller 46 Versuchstage 9 ± 3 % betrug.

Durch Berücksichtigung des ermittelten Zusammenhanges zwischen Wärmeproduktion und MSA konnte eine Reduzierung der Standardabweichung der täglichen Wärmeproduktion um 44 % bei der Ratte und um 33 % beim Schwein erreicht werden.

СОДЕРЖАНИЕ

INHALT

ARCHIVES OF ANIMAL NUTRITION
ARCHIV FÜR TIERERNÄHRUNG

VOLUME 37 OCTOBER 1987 NUMBER 10

CONTENTS

Archives of Animal Nutrition is indexed in Current Contents Agriculture, Biology & Environmental Sciences, and abstracted in Nutrition Abstracts & Review and in Chemical Abstracts.

Bei Fragen zur Produktsicherheit wenden Sie sich bitte an:
If you have any questions regarding product safety,
please contact:

Walter de Gruyter GmbH
Genthiner Straße 13
10785 Berlin
productsafety@degruyterbrill.com